Counseling & Diversity

Counseling Asian Americans

Counseling & Diversity

Counseling Asian Americans

Bryan S. K. Kim
University of Hawai'i at Hilo

Series Editors
Azara Santiago-Rivera and Devika Dibya Choudhuri

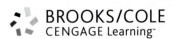
BROOKS/COLE
CENGAGE Learning™

Australia • Brazil • Japan • Korea • Mexico • Singapore • Spain • United Kingdom • United States

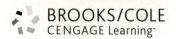

**Counseling & Diversity: Counseling
Asian Americans**
Bryan S. K. Kim

Series Editors: Azara Santiago-Rivera and
Devika Dibya Choudhuri

Acquisitions Editor: Seth Dobrin

Assistant Editor: Nicolas Albert

Editorial Assistant: Rachel McDonald

Marketing Manager: Trent Whatcott

Production Manager: Matt Ballantyne

Art Director: Caryl Gorska

Print Buyer: Paula Vang

Rights Acquisitions Account Manager, Text:
Bob Kauser

Cover Image: Getty/Thinkstock Images

Compositor: Pre-PressPMG

For more information about our products, contact us at:
Cengage Learning Customer Sales & Support, 1-800-354-9706

For permission to use material from this text or product,
submit a request online at **www.cengage.com/permissions**
Further permissions can be emailed to
permissionrequest@cengage.com

Library of Congress Control Number: 2010922112
ISBN-13: 978-0-618-47037-2
ISBN-10: 0-618-47037-9

Brooks/Cole
20 Davis Drive
Belmont, CA 94002-3098
USA

Cengage Learning is a leading provider of customized learning solutions with
office locations around the globe, including Singapore, the United Kingdom,
Australia, Mexico, Brazil, and Japan. Locate your local office at:
international.cengage.com/region

Cengage Learning products are represented in Canada by
Nelson Education, Ltd.

For your course and learning solutions, visit **academic.cengage.com**

Printed in the United States of America
1 2 3 4 5 6 7 14 13 12 11 10

CONTENTS

To Robyn, Sydney, and Courtney – the wonderful girls in my life.

Introduction

Welcome! I feel honored and privileged to have this opportunity to share with you information about culturally competent counseling with Asian-American clients. Asian Americans represent one of the fastest growing cultural groups in the United States. For example, between 1990 and 2000 the number of Asian Americans increased by 72%, and as of 2007, Asian Americans numbered 15.2 million or 5% of the total U.S. population (Barnes & Bennett, 2002). By 2050, it is estimated that one out of every 10 Americans in the United States will have an Asian ancestry. This rapid growth in size, combined with research data showing that Asian Americans tend to underutilize counseling services, although their need for these services is no less than other groups, has led to an increased attention by mental health professionals. One area of attention has been to train counselors to have competence in providing culturally relevant, sensitive, and effective services to clients from this significant segment of the U.S. population. Given that you are reading this book, I assume that you are a part of this group of counselors who are interested in increasing their effectiveness with Asian-American clients. I hope the information contained in this volume will serve you well as you embark on your journey to becoming an expert in working with this unique and growing population.

In this book, I will present various issues related to effective counseling with Asian-American clients. My working thesis is that having a good understanding of the demographic, historical, sociopolitical, and cultural characteristics of Asian Americans will increase the likelihood of counselors implementing more relevant and effective services with this population. It is my belief that culturally competent counseling with Asian Americans goes beyond just learning some recipe of strategies, but includes a more thorough understanding of the overall psychological characteristics of Asian Americans. Therefore, the major goals of the book are for you to gain an in-depth understanding about the following topics related to the experiences of Asian Americans: (a) demographic profile, (b) sociopolitical history, (c) current status regarding oppression and resiliency, (d) cultural systems, and (e) counseling dynamics and interventions. As you read the book, I would like you to keep in mind the following questions: Who are Asian Americans? How have their psychological experiences been shaped by external factors such as history and culture? and what implications does this information have for you as a counselor who will be working with these individuals? This inquisitive attitude could serve you well as you try to understand the nature of Asian-American clients.

Now, allow me share a little bit about myself so that you have an idea of where I am coming from. It is my belief that any writing, including that based on factual information, is inherently influenced by the worldview of its author. In brief, *worldview* refers to attitudes and beliefs one has about the nature and function of the world, and is influenced by one's cultural socialization. Hence, I believe all writings to reflect, to one degree or another, the authors' own unique views about what is true about the world. As you read the book, you might be able to see that, indeed for me too, the writings are influenced by my own worldview, including my biases and prejudices. So that you can be clear about these influences, allow me to describe the process of socialization that contributed to my own worldview.

I am a 1.5-generation Asian American, more specifically a Korean American, who immigrated to the United States at the age of nine years. I arrived in Hawai'i in 1979 and lived there until I went to California in 1996 to work on my doctorate. Consequently, much of my identity as an Asian American stems from my experiences growing up in Hawai'i, a place of immense ethnic and cultural diversity. For instance, Hawai'i has the largest percentage of people with a multiracial and multiethnic background in the United States. Growing up in Hawai'i allowed me to not only experience the tensions and joys related to diversity, but more importantly, to see how people who are multiculturally competent learn to thrive in this environment. A more formal education in diversity occurred while I earned a bachelor's degree in science education and a master's degree in school counseling from the University of Hawai'i at Manoa. During this time, I was fortunate to have worked with professors who introduced me to the field of multicultural counseling. My education in diversity continued when I was admitted to the Counseling, Clinical, and School Psychology Program (with a Counseling Psychology emphasis) at the University of California, Santa Barbara. With expert guidance and mentoring from the faculty at UCSB (particularly my advisor, the late Professor Emeritus Donald R. Atkinson), my interest in multiculturalism and counseling competence grew and became more formalized. In essence, this is where I gained a more disciplined understanding about the nature of cultural diversity vis-à-vis counseling, psychology, and education. (However, this is not to imply that any shortcomings in this book should be attributed to my former teachers and mentors.)

After finishing my coursework and dissertation at UCSB in 1999, I went to live in Fort Collins, Colorado, for my pre-doctoral internship at Colorado State University. After completing the one-year internship, I was hired as a tenure-track assistant professor of counseling psychology at the University of Maryland in College Park. After two years, I returned to UCSB as a tenure-track assistant professor. After earning tenure and promotion to associate professor at UCSB, I returned to Hawai'i in 2006 to join the faculty at the University of Hawai'i at Hilo's counseling psychology program and became its director in 2008. Given all of these travels across the country and back, I was able to further gain both personal and intellectual lessons about how diversity manifests itself in the various parts of the United States and how people in these regions are coping with and even thriving in it. At the present time, my research is focused on the experiences of Asian Americans around the issues of multicultural counseling process and outcome, measurement of cultural constructs, counselor education and supervision, and immigrant experiences.

I want to thank the editors of this series, Drs. Azara Santiago-Rivera and Devika Dibya Choudhuri, the former Senior Editor at Lahaska Press/ Houghton Mifflin, Ms. Mary Falcon, the Helping Professions Acquisitions Editor at Cengage, Mr. Seth Dobrin, and the Counseling Assistant Editor at Cengage, Mr. Nicolas Albert, for giving me this opportunity to share my thoughts about counseling Asian Americans and for their excellent guidance and support throughout the process of writing this volume. In addition, I want to thank Dr. Allen Ivey who introduced me to Lahaska Press that led to my involvement in this project.

To conclude, I hope you will find the information in this book useful. If you have any comments or questions, please feel free to contact me at bryankim@hawaii.edu.

Aloha,
BSKK

Counseling & Diversity

Counseling Asian Americans

CHAPTER 1

A Demographic Profile of Asian Americans

This chapter provides a description of Asian Americans in the United States in terms of their demographic characteristics. As you read this chapter, I invite you to consider the following questions.

- What are the numerical size of the Asian-American population, their Asian ethnic backgrounds, and their age range?

- What are Asian-Americans' immigration patterns and geographical settlement areas?

- What are Asian-Americans' educational attainments, income and family composition, poverty rate, and employment outcome?

POPULATION SIZE

During the last four decades, the Asian-American population has been one of the fastest growing groups in the United States. As of the last U.S. census in 2000, the number of Asian Americans stood at nearly 4.2% of the total U.S. population (see Table 1; Barnes & Bennett, 2002). In comparison to the 1990 census figure, there were 5 million more persons reporting an Asian ancestry, representing an increase of more than 70% (Gibson & Jung, 2002).

TABLE **1**

Demographic Characteristics of Asian Americans

Population Size by Year (Percentage of Total U.S. population)			
1970	1980	1990	2000
1.5 million	3.5 million	6.9 million	11.9 million
(0.8%)	(1.5%)	(2.8%)	(4.2%)

Percentage of Total Asian American Population by Age Range in Years						
Under 5	5 to 13	14 to 17	18 to 24	25 to 44	45 to 64	Over 65
7.4%	12.7%	5.6%	11.0%	34.8%	20.4%	8.1%

Largest Groups of Asian Immigrants in Percentage of Total U.S. Immigrant Population				
Ethnic Chinese	Filipinos	Asian Indians	Vietnamese	Koreans
4.9%	4.4%	3.3%	3.2%	2.8%

Geographical Settlement Areas in Percentage of Total Asian American Population			
Western States	Northeast States	Southern States	Midwestern States
49%	20%	19%	12%

Educational Attainment in Percentage of Total Asian American Population (Average for European Americans)			
High School	Some College	Bachelor's Degree	Advanced Degree
80.4% (85.5%)	64.6% (55.4%)	44.1% (27.0%)	17.4% (9.8%)

Family Income in Percentage of Total Asian American (and Pacific Islander) Population (Average for European Americans)				
Below $25000	$25000–$34999	$35000–$49999	$50000–$74999	$75000 and Over
14.3% (11.8%)	7.4% (9.6%)	13.5% (15.0%)	20.6% (23.5%)	44.2% (40.1%)

Poverty Status by Age in Percentage of Total Asian American (and Pacific Islander) Population (Average for European Americans)		
Under 18 Years	18 to 64 Years	65 Years and Over
11.5% (9.5%)	9.7% (7.2%)	10.2% (8.1%)

To further illustrate the dramatic increase of this population, Asian Americans in 1980 and 1970 made up only 1.5% and 0.8%, respectively, of the total U.S. population (Gibson & Jung, 2002). This rapid growth of Asian Americans is projected to continue into the next several decades. Currently, Asian Americans make up 15.2 million individuals representing 5% of the total U.S. population (U.S. Bureau of Census, 2009). By 2050, it is estimated that one out of 10 people living in the United States will be able to trace their ancestry in part or full to Asian countries (U.S. Bureau of Census, 2004).

One obvious implication stemming from these statistics is that professional counselors across the United States will see an increasing number of Asian Americans in their work settings. Thus it is critical for counselors to familiarize themselves with the psychological characteristics of Asian Americans and how counselors can be more culturally relevant, sensitive, and effective with this significant segment of our population.

ETHNIC BACKGROUND

The Asian-American population represents a very heterogeneous group representing many ethnic backgrounds that have distinct cultural norms. Although they have been classified as a single group because of their common geographical origins on the Asian continent, the group includes over two dozen sub-ethnic groups. Shown in Table 2 is the list of Asian ethnic groups and their numbers based on the 2000 U.S. census. As you can see, the Asian-American group includes individuals from a wide range of geographical origins, including East Asian countries, such as China and Japan; Southeast Asian countries, such as Vietnam, Philippines, and Indonesia; and South Asian countries, such as India and Pakistan. In terms of number, Chinese represent the numerically largest group, followed by Filipinos, Asian Indians, Koreans, Vietnamese, and Japanese, with all of these groups having at least one million individuals. As with their countries of origin, these ethnic groups, which are represented under the rubric of Asian American, also vary significantly in their language, traditions, customs, societal norms, and immigration history.

As you are reviewing this population data, it is important to keep in mind that in the past the U.S. Bureau of Census utilized various definitions of the Asian-American group. For instance, previous to 1980, Asian Indians were not counted as part of Asian Americans but were considered a part of the white group. Until 2000, Asian Americans were grouped with Pacific Islanders; the most recent census reported separate population counts for these groups. Also until 2000, multiracial Asian Americans (i.e., individuals who can trace their ancestry to one or more other racial groups in addition to Asian American) were not allowed to indicate more than one race, leading to a possible undercount of Asian Americans; in 2000, there were 1.7 million (0.6% of total population) multiracial Asian Americans (see Table 2).

Despite the varying definitions of who comprise Asian Americans, what is clear is that Asian Americans make up a very heterogeneous group of people.

TABLE **2**
Asian American Population by Ethnicity

Asian Ethnicity	Asian Ethnicity Alone		Asian Ethnicity in Combination with One or More Other Races		Either Asian Alone or in Any Combination of Race and Ethnicity
	One Asian Ethnicity Reported	More Than One Asian Ethnicity Reported	One Asian Ethnicity Reported	More Than One Asian Ethnicity Reported	
TOTAL	10,019,405	223,593	1,516,841	138,989	11,898,828
Asian Indian	1,678,765	40,013	165,437	15,384	1,899,599
Bangladeshi	41,280	5,625	9,655	852	57,412
Bhutanese	183	9	17	3	212
Burmese	13,159	1,461	1,837	263	16,720
Cambodian	171,937	11,832	20,830	1,453	206,052
Chinese, except Taiwanese	2,314,537	130,826	201,688	87,790	2,734,841
Filipino	1,850,314	57,811	385,236	71,454	2,364,815
Hmong	169,428	5,284	11,153	445	186,310
Indo Chinese	133	55	23	8	199
Indonesian	39,757	4,429	17,256	1,631	63,073

Iwo Jiman	15	3	60	–	78
Japanese	796,700	55,537	241,209	55,486	1,148,932
Korean	1,076,872	22,550	114,211	14,794	1,228,427
Laotian	168,707	10,396	17,914	1,186	198,203
Malaysian	10,690	4,339	2,837	700	18,566
Maldivian	27	2	22	–	51
Nepalese	7,858	351	1,128	62	9,399
Okinawan	3,513	2,625	2,816	1,645	10,599
Pakistani	153,533	11,095	37,587	2,094	204,309
Singaporean	1,437	580	307	70	2,394
Sri Lankan	20,145	1,219	2,966	257	24,587
Taiwanese	118,048	14,096	11,394	1,257	144,795
Thai	112,989	7,929	27,170	2,195	150,283
Vietnamese	1,122,528	47,144	48,639	5,425	1,223,736
Other Asian ethnicity	146,870	19,576	195,449	7,535	369,430

Adapted from Barnes and Bennett (2002).

What may also be clear is that effective counseling with Asian Americans requires an appreciation for this wide range of ethnic diversity and the resulting differences in cultural norms. Indeed, gaining an accurate understanding of within-group variations may represent a significant challenge for professional counselors working with Asian Americans, and it will be one of the major foci of this book.

AGE RANGE

According to the 2000 U.S. census, Asian Americans in general with a median age of 31.1 years tend to be younger than the rest of the population whose median age was 35.3 years (U.S. Bureau of the Census, 2002). As shown in Table 1, about 35% of Asian Americans were between the ages of 25 and 44 years. The second largest group of Asian Americans was under the age of 18, comprising about 25% and with half of this group between the ages of 5 and 13 years. A group in the age range of 45 to 64 years, making up about 20% of the population, followed this group.

Based on these numbers, it is reasonable to hypothesize that counselors probably will encounter Asian-American clients in different age brackets whose counseling needs will vary. Similar to ethnic variations, counselors should become familiar with the unique needs of these individuals to provide effective counseling. For example, one of the important implications in working with younger Asian Americans is to deal with acculturation gaps between themselves and their parents, which could lead to intergenerational conflicts. For older Asian Americans who immigrated to this country, they may experience difficulties related to missing their friends and similar-age relatives in their countries of origin. I will discuss more about these issues later in the book.

IMMIGRATION PATTERN

This dramatic increase in the number of Asian Americans is largely a result of the huge influx of immigrants from Asia. As of 2000, there were over 8.2 million Asian Americans in the United States who were born in Asia, representing nearly seven of 10 Asian Americans (Malone, Baluja, Costanzo, & Davis, 2003). In comparison to other racial groups, these Asian Americans made up over one-quarter (26.4%) of the total number of foreign-born Americans, a significant percentage when considering that Asian Americans made up 4.2% of the U.S. population in 2000. In terms of specific Asian countries of origin, the 2000 census indicated that the combined numbers of migrants from China, Hong Kong, Taiwan, and the Paracel Islands (categorized as the Ethnic Chinese group in Table 1) had the second highest percentage (after Mexico) of foreign-born Americans. China was followed by the Philippines, India, Vietnam, and Korea. In total, these five Asian countries accounted for a total of 5.8 million Asian migrants to the United States (see Table 1).

Given this high number of immigrants within the Asian-American population, counselors will have to deal with the fact that for many of these individuals English will be a second language and they will be experiencing difficulties in adjusting to their new lives in the United States. Furthermore, many of these individuals may not be familiar with conventional forms of counseling, or even if they do, they may not know where and how to seek help. To meet these needs, counselors must become more familiar with these and other challenges facing these people and ways to appropriately address them.

GEOGRAPHICAL SETTLEMENT AREAS

Asian Americans reside in various locations across the United States, with nearly half of them living in the Western states, followed by the states in the Northeast, South, and Midwest (see Table 1; Barnes & Bennett, 2002). As of the 2000 census, California had the highest number of Asian Americans with 4.2 million, making up 12.3% of the state population. New York was a distant second with 1.2 million, making up 6.2% of the state population. Hawai'i was third with 0.7 million, although making up 58% of the state population. Interestingly, almost three out of 10 Asian Americans in Hawai'i reported one or more other race indicating the presence of a high rate of multiracial Asian Americans. The number of Asian Americans in these three states represented just over half (51%) of the total Asian population, although these states accounted for just 19% of the total U.S. population. Other states that have high numbers of Asian Americans are, in ranked order: Texas, New Jersey, Illinois, Washington, and Florida.

As shown here, Asian Americans live all across the United States but vary in their percentages from state to state. Hence, counselors must understand the degree to which these individuals are impacted by their minority status relative to the percentage of majority population and access to their ethnic enclaves. For example, Asian Americans living in a rural town in Iowa will certainly have different counseling needs in comparison to their counterparts living in San Francisco's Chinatown where they comprise a large and visible segment of the city population.

EDUCATIONAL ATTAINMENT

In general, Asian Americans tend to be a well-educated group (Bauman & Graf, 2003). In comparison to European Americans and other racial groups, Asian Americans in 2000 had higher levels of educational attainment in attending college and earning a bachelor's or advanced degrees (see Table 1). Eight of 10 Asian Americans have completed high school, a figure that was only second to the graduation rate of European Americans (see Table 1). However, there is also evidence suggesting that many Asian Americans significantly deviate from these positive trends. In a recent study comparing Asian Americans and Pacific Islanders as a whole with European Americans (Pacific Islanders make up 0.3% of the population so one could reason that these figures are largely representative of Asian Americans), Reeves and Bennett (2003) found that Asian Americans and Pacific Islanders were almost twice as likely to have less than a ninth-grade education than European Americans; 7% for Asian Americans and Pacific Islanders vs. 4% for European Americans. Also, given the large number of Asian Americans who were born outside of the United States, there are many individuals who are not proficient in the English language, which could impede their educational attainment in the United States. Furthermore, there are significant variations among the various Asian-American ethnic groups in terms of educational attainment. While groups such as Asian Indians, Chinese, and Japanese tend to have higher rates of educational attainment than European Americans, other Asian Americans such as Cambodian, Hmong, and Vietnamese tend to be underrepresented in this group (Hsia & Peng, 1998).

These figures show the presence of significant within group variations across the various Asian-American groups in terms of educational attainment. Thus, counselors must be careful to not assume that all Asian Americans have fared well in our educational system and must be sensitive to the varying educational needs of these individuals. I will discuss more about this issue later in the book when describing the model minority myth.

INCOME AND FAMILY COMPOSITION

Paralleling the ethnic diversity on the rates of educational attainment, there is a significant variation in the amount of income for Asian-American families. On the high end, there were more Asian-American (and Pacific Islander) families in 2001 who earned $75,000 or more per year than European-American families (Reeves & Bennett, 2003). However, at the low end of the spectrum, more Asian-American (and Pacific-Islander) families in 2001 earned less than $25,000 than European-American families. Also, the figures at the high end of the spectrum must be considered within the context of family size. The higher-than-average family income for Asian Americans may be an attributed to more people working to contribute to the family's earnings. In 2002, 19.9% of Asian Americans lived in families with five or more members, whereas the same statistic was 12.1% for European Americans (Reeves & Bennett, 2003). For a family of four members, 27% of Asian Americans lived in such a setting, whereas 21.2% of European Americans lived in a family of four. Consistent with these trends, a more recent estimate showed that the median per capita income for Asian Americans was $29,901, whereas for European Americans it was $31,051 (DeNavas-Walt, Proctor, & Smith, 2008).

An important implication of this conclusion is that there may be structural and societal injustices in terms of how much Asian Americans as individuals may earn in comparison to European Americans. Also, counselors should keep in mind that not all Asian-American families are doing well financially. As you will see in the next paragraph, this is clearly evident in the Asian-Americans' rates of poverty.

POVERTY RATE

Corresponding to income statistics, there is also a significant discrepancy in the percentage of Asian Americans living in poverty in comparison to European Americans. According to Reeves and Bennett (2003), 10.2% of Asian Americans, or 1.3 million, lived in poverty, whereas the same figure is 7.8% for European Americans. In a more recent estimate, the poverty rate for Asian Americans remained the same at 10.2%, whereas the rate for European

Americans increased slightly to 8.2% (DeNavas-Walt, Proctor, & Smith, 2008). As shown in Table 1, this group of Asian Americans includes a high percentage of the elderly population, who tend to have low-paying and low (low-status) jobs as compared to those in the European-American population (Wong & Ujimoto, 1998). In addition, there is an overrepresentation of Southeast Asians in this group suffering from poverty. While the national poverty rate in 1995 was 13.1%, Cambodian-American, Vietnamese-American, Laotian-American, and Hmong-American groups had the following percentages: 42.6%, 25.7%, 34.7%, and 63.6%, respectively (Rumbaut, 1995).

An important implication for counselors is that they need to be aware that many Asian Americans are not faring well in the United States. Counselors will need to be prepared to address issues of poverty, particularly among significant segments of the Asian-American population such as the elderly and some Southeast Asian groups.

EMPLOYMENT OUTCOME

In terms of occupations, Asian Americans are employed in a wide range of positions. In 2002, 39.1% of Asian Americans occupied managerial and professional positions, a percentage that was higher than that for European Americans (35.2%). For other positions, the percentages between the two groups were comparable, with the statistic for Asian Americans being 28.2% in technical, sales, and administrative support positions and 14.6% in service positions. These findings have important implications particularly for career counselors. For example, these counselors must be aware of the types of occupations and careers that are occupied by Asian Americans, but careful of not pigeon-holing these individuals to a narrow array of possible jobs.

SUMMARY AND CONCLUSIONS

As described here, Asian Americans represent a very fast-growing group with tremendous diversity. They represent over 25 ethnic groups with different language, cultural customs, and traditions (see Table 2 for a listing of these groups). Asian Americans tend to live all across the United States, but particularly in California, New York, and Hawai'i. Asian Americans tend to be a young, well-educated group, although there are important variations within the group with many individuals who are not able to obtain a high level of education. In addition, although many Asian-American families earn more than European-American families, this finding is tempered by the fact that the median per capita income for Asian Americans tends to be less than that of European Americans and that Asian Americans are overrepresented among those living in poverty. Finally, Asian Americans occupy various positions in the civilian labor force.

All of these descriptions point to the fact that Asian Americans represent a highly diverse population with significant variations on many demographic characteristics. To meet the unique needs that arise from this diversity, counselors must first become knowledgeable about the historical, social, and political bases for these variations. The next chapter will address these issues.

CHAPTER 2

A Sociopolitical History of Asian Americans

Just as there is tremendous ethnic diversity within the Asian American population, there are significant variations on the immigration histories of Asian Americans. In this section, I present a description of Asian American immigration into the United States, starting in the mid-1800s and continuing to the present time. I also highlight various social and political issues within each time period that have had an impact on the status of Asian Americans. As I mentioned earlier, it is my thesis that an accurate understanding of Asian American history is critical to providing relevant and effective counseling services to Asian Americans. As you read this section, please consider the following questions.

- How did different groups of Asian Americans arrive in the United States? What were their immediate and long-term experiences?

- How did various social trends and governmental policies affect the lives of Asian Americans?

- How have Asian Americans proven their validity as Americans?

1848 TO 1924: THE FIRST ARRIVALS

The presence of Asians in North America can be traced to Filipino sailors, known as "Manilamen," who settled in the areas around Louisiana in the mid-1500s (Chan, 1991). However, the first large wave of migration from Asia to the United States did not begin until 1848 with the arrival of Chinese laborers from Southern China to San Francisco (Chan, 1991; Wong, 1998). The Chinese were soon followed by Japanese migrants in 1868, Koreans in 1903, and Filipinos in 1906, most of whom initially entered Hawai'i to work on its sugar plantations (Chan, 1991). Asian Indians began arriving in 1907 to work on the railroads and the agricultural fields of California.

After hearing about the discovery of gold in California, the first large groups of Chinese began to arrive in San Francisco in 1848 (Chan, 1991). In 1852 alone, more than 20,000 Chinese sailed into San Francisco harbor headed for the gold fields in the Sierra Nevada foothills (Chan, 1991). Another group of more than 40,000 Chinese entered the United States between 1867 and 1870. However, as their numbers continued to grow, so did the prejudice and discrimination against them (Chan, 1991). Many Americans during the nineteenth century viewed the Chinese as "nothing more than starving masses, beasts of burden, depraved heathens, and opium addicts" (Chan, 1991, p. 45).

Fueled by these negative views, a number of discriminatory legislations were passed against the Chinese. One of the more outrageous laws was enacted by the San Francisco Board of Supervisors in 1870. In this law, laundry vendors using one horse for their delivery wagons had to pay two dollars every three months, those using two horses paid four dollars, while those using no horses were charged fifteen dollars. Because laundry vendors who did not use horses were mainly the Chinese, the law in effect was targeted on them (Chan, 1991). Also, Chinese were targets of physical violence (Chan, 1991). For example, in 1885 in Rock Springs in the Wyoming Territory, a group of striking white workers attacked and killed 28 Chinese and wounded 15 more who refused to join the strike. These anti-Chinese sentiments finally culminated in the passing of the Chinese Exclusion Act in 1882 that forbade any more Chinese laborers from entering the United States.

In addition to these discriminatory acts, Chinese laborers also suffered from a lack of connection to or support from any family ties in the United States. The laborers were largely comprised of single men who entered the United States alone and whose hopes were to return to China after a few years. Even among those men who had wives and children in China, they did not bring their families to the United States because they also intended to return to China in a short time. In fact, out of almost 90,000 Chinese on the U.S. mainland in 1900, only 5% were female (many of these women were brought to the United States to serve as prostitutes for the laborers) (Takaki, 1989). However, given the difficulties of barely earning enough money to survive, most of the laborers were not able to return to China, while the laborers who were able to return did so without the fortune they expected to have made. Also, even if the laborers made enough money to bring their wives to the United States, a ruling by the Circuit Court of California in 1884 (*In Re Ah*

Moy, on Habeas Corpus), two years after the passing of the Chinese Exclusion Act, denied entrance to wives of Chinese residents in the United States (Takaki, 1989). Consequently, these factors led to the creation of a large community of Chinese men who had no families.

Fortunately for some of these men who lived in San Francisco, a door for Chinese women to enter the United States was opened in 1906 when an earthquake hit the city and destroyed almost all of the municipal records. Many of the Chinese laborers whose records were destroyed could now claim that they had been born in the United States, and as citizens they could bring wives and children into the United States. As a result, the number of Chinese women who entered the United States between 1907 and 1924 increased dramatically to about 10,000, representing about one-quarter of all Chinese immigrants (Takaki, 1989). This increase in number eventually led to having about 20% women among the Chinese population. Among the rest of the immigrants from China, most were children who suddenly became U.S. citizens when their fathers became citizens. Also among this group were some "paper sons" who had purchased birth certificates of these American citizens born in China and then claimed their citizenship to enter the United States (Takaki, 1989).

Aside from Chinese migration to California, there also were many Chinese who migrated to Hawai'i to work in the sugar plantations (Chan, 1991; Takaki, 1983). Sugar played a major economic role in Hawai'i beginning in the mid-1850s when foreigners bought large chunks of real estate and began to harvest sugar cane that grew well in the volcanic soils and the year-round warm climate. Fueling this new industry was a large market in the world for sugar, particularly in the United States whose sugar production had been decimated by the Civil War. This situation created a demand that the sugar planters very much wanted to meet and, because sugarcane cultivation is highly labor intensive, the planters became desperate for cheap sources of manual labor (Chan, 1991; Takaki, 1983). However, the diseases introduced by foreigners such as smallpox, syphilis, and tuberculosis decimated the native Hawai'ian population. When Captain James Cook arrived in the Hawai'i islands in 1778, there were approximately one million native Hawai'ians. But by the 1890s, this number dropped to 40,000. Hence, there were no other viable sources of workers in Hawai'i. Given this predicament, the sugar planters turned to foreign countries, particularly in Asia. Upon hearing that the Chinese were good farm workers, the sugar planters first recruited workers from China. As a result, while only 151 Chinese entered Hawai'i in 1875, 1,283 did so in 1876. Altogether, approximately 50,000 Chinese entered Hawai'i between 1852 and the end of the nineteenth century (Chan, 1991).

However, by the 1880s, the sugar planters also faced the growing anti-Chinese sentiments and the push toward barring immigration of Chinese workers. Hawai'i became a territory of the United States in 1900 and the Chinese Exclusion Act became law in the islands at this time. As a result, the planters sought to recruit workers from other Asian countries, and in particular, Japan. The first group of Japanese laborers arrived in 1885, and the Japanese population reached its peak between 1894 and 1908 when about 125,000 Japanese workers migrated to Hawai'i (Chan, 1991). However, as a result of anti-Japanese sentiments on the mainland and some in Hawai'i that were fueled by notions such as "yellow peril" and "unassimilable aliens," the U.S. government convinced the Japanese government to ban emigration of its citizens into the United States. Consequently, Japanese immigration to the United States, including Hawai'i, ended in 1908 with the signing of the 1907 Gentlemen's Agreement between the governments of United States and Japan (Takaki, 1983).

But even before the signing of the 1907 Agreement, the sugar planters had become wary of the growing number of Japanese workers and the possibility of the workers organizing to form a labor union and so they began to look for other sources of cheap labor (Patterson, 1988). Upon hearing from missionaries stationed in Korea, that Koreans were "docile workers," the sugar planters successfully made arrangements to import workers from Korea and the first shipload of Korean workers arrived in Hawai'i in January 1903. The migration of Korean workers ended abruptly in 1905 when the Japanese government, upon hearing that Korean workers were being used as strike breakers against Japanese workers who were striking, forced the Korean king to prohibit further emigration of Korean workers to Hawai'i. As a result, only a total of 6,747 Korean workers entered the United States during this three-year period (Patterson, 1988). However, Korean immigration was not completely suspended as approximately 1,000 picture brides and 900 political exiles entered the United States between 1910 and 1924.

The banning of immigration from China, Japan, and Korea created an urgent need for a new source of workers for the sugar planters. The planters turned to the Philippines as the new source of labor (Espiritu, 1995). Because the Philippines were at that time a territory of the United States, Filipinos were considered U.S. nationals and could freely travel to the United States. In addition, many Filipinos were able to serve in the U.S. Navy, which allowed them to travel to the United States easily. Filipinos were the only Asians who served in the U.S. military in sizable numbers without holding U.S. citizenship. Between 1907 and 1935, 122, 100 Filipinos arrived in Hawai'i.

Early migration of Asian Indians to the United States took a different route. Most Asian Indians initially entered Canada as subjects of the British Empire (Jensen, 1988). However, not unlike the Asians living in the United States, they faced prejudice and discrimination from Canadians (Jensen, 1988). Finally, as a result of anti-Indian violence, many Asian Indians migrated south into the United States, first to Washington and then finally to California to work in farms and the railroad industry. A total of about 7,000 Asian Indians migrated to the United States in the early 1900s.

In general, the continued entry and the increasing number of Asians further fueled anti-Asian sentiments (Chan, 1991). In the eyes of many, including the U.S. Supreme Court, Asians were seen as "unassimilable aliens" who could not become part of the society. As a result, Asians could not become naturalized citizens (e.g., Naturalization Act of 1870), Asians were not allowed to own land (1913 California Alien Land Law), and white women who married Asian men were forced to give up their citizenship (1905 California Anti-Miscegenation Law, 1922 U.S. Cable Act). Interestingly, Asian Indians, because they were of the Caucasoid race and did not look "oriental," were granted citizenship in some states, but only until the U.S. Supreme Court in the case of United States v. Bhagat Singh Thind (1923) determined that Asian Indians did not qualify to be citizens (Chan, 1991). This decision was significant in that it changed the previous biological race-based criterion to a more arbitrary socially constructed definition of being white and a U.S. citizen.

The influx of millions of Southern European migrants into the United States gave further cause for the U.S. public to become even more hostile toward immigration. Finally, the U.S. Congress passed the Immigration Act of 1924 that virtually ended all migration into the United States from Asia and Southern Europe. Despite all of this resistance, however, approximately one million Asians entered the United States between 1848 and 1924 (Chan, 1991).

1924 TO 1965: THE SECOND ARRIVALS AND JAPANESE INTERNMENT

Although immigration from Asia was severely curtailed by the Immigration Act of 1924, several thousand Asians were able to enter the United States between 1924 and 1965. Most of these individuals were wives of military soldiers stationed in various Asian countries during World War II (1941–1945) and the Korean War (1950–1953) (Chan, 1991). These wives tended to fall into two categories: those who married other Asians and those who married non-Asians. For the first category, approximately 9,000 Chinese women entered the United States after marrying Chinese American soldiers. Japanese, Korean, and Filipina women tended to marry European American soldiers. Between 2,000 and 5,000 Japanese women entered the United States per year in the 1950s and the early 1960s. In the 1950s, about 500 Korean women arrived annually as wives of U.S. soldiers who were stationed there. This number increased to about 1,500 per year in the early 1960's. As for Filipina wives, about 1,000 women arrived annually in the 1950s and this number rose to about 1,500 per year in the 1960s (Chan, 1991).

Japanese Internment

While the U.S. government made some positive changes to the highly restrictive immigration policy, the government at the start of World War II also engaged in an egregious act of uprooting and detaining all Japanese Americans living in the West Coast. Soon after the December 7, 1941 Japanese attack on Pearl Harbor, General John L. DeWitt, commander of the Western Defense Command and under the authority granted him by Executive Order 9066, forcefully interned 112,000 Japanese living on the Pacific Coast, including thousands of U.S.-born citizens, into 10 "relocation centers" (also known as internment camps) in desolate areas of California, Idaho, Wyoming, Utah, Arizona, Colorado, and Arkansas (Spickard, 1996). The U.S. political leaders believed that Japanese Americans would forever be loyal to the Emperor of Japan, would support the Japanese war effort by sabotaging important infrastructures in the West Coast, and could not be trusted to be loyal to the United States. All of these beliefs were without any tangible evidence.

Before relocating to the camps for the duration of the war, the Japanese Americans were forced to give up most of their material possessions, including their houses, businesses, and land. Upon arrival at the camps, Japanese Americans who had lived lives of self-reliance and independence suddenly became completely dependent on the government for work, food, and housing (Takaki, 1989). They could not leave the camps and were guarded around the clock by armed U.S. soldiers.

The basic living conditions also were dreadful. Each family of four to six persons shared a room measuring 20 feet by 25 feet without any furniture. All of the internees had to share communal bathrooms with no partitions, and there were constant complaints about the food (Chan, 1991). Also, the family structure began to deteriorate in the camps. The authority and status of the fathers began to erode when they lost their role as the leading breadwinner. Consequently, the children often ate meals with their friends rather than their families and roamed the center without parental control. [To learn more about the experiences of Japanese Americans during this time, consider viewing "Children of the Camps" (Ina, 1999) a video documentary about six Japanese Americans who were interned as children and their struggles during and after this experience.]

Amazingly, only the Japanese Americans living on the U.S. mainland were targeted for relocation, and the large numbers of Americans whose ancestries trace to Germany and Italy, the two countries who also were at war with the United States, were spared of this forced imprisonment. Also ironically, the 442nd Regimental Combat Team, which was comprised of Nisei Japanese Americans, many of whom were interned at relocation camps, proved their loyalty to the United States by becoming the most decorated unit of its size during World War II. By the end of the war, this unit suffered 9,486 casualties, including 600 killed (Takaki, 1989). They earned over 18,000 individual decorations including one Congressional Medal of Honor, 47 Distinguished Service Crosses, 350 Silver Stars, 810 Bronze Stars, and over 3,600 Purple Hearts (Takaki, 1989).

Finally, in 1988, acknowledging this clear act of injustice to Japanese Americans, the U.S. government agreed to make a formal apology and pay $20,000 in reparation to each individual who was interned (Spickard, 1996). Similarly, the University of California in 2009 granted honorary degrees to approximately 700 Japanese Americans students at its Berkeley, Davis, Los Angeles, and San Francisco campuses who were interned in 1942 and could not complete their college education (Your University of California Online, 2009).

1965 TO THE PRESENT: THE IMMIGRATION ACT OF 1965

The 1960s was a tumultuous time in U.S. history. The social and political landscape was in a major upheaval as many Americans, and racial minorities in particular, engaged in a fight for equality and justice. Asian Americans, which included mainly the second, third, and fourth generation descendants of the earlier immigrants, were significant and visible participants in this effort. One major outcome of their work is the formation of a pan-Asian ethnic identity, which changed the identity of various Asian ethnic groups into the collective "Asian Americans" (Wei, 1993). The leaders of this movement realized that the notion of an Asian American identity could bring together the members of varied Asian ethnic groups and allow them to have greater social and political voice in the United States. This effort to increase the visibility of Asian Americans took a giant leap forward with the arrival of significant numbers of Asians into the United States after the passing of the 1965 Immigration Act.

Immigration Act of 1965

One of the significant outcomes of the Civil Rights Movement is the passing of the Immigration Act of 1965 by the U.S. Congress. This Act represented an attempt to change the international image of the United States as a leading country committed to freedom, equality, and justice; previous to it, the severe immigration restrictions imposed by the 1924 Immigration Act hindered the development of this image. The 1965 Act (and the 1990 extension of that Act) had the following two goals: family reunification and importation of skilled workers (Ong, & Liu, 1994). The goal of reunifying family members resulted in giving immigration priority to persons who were joining their families already residing in the United States. The goal of importing skilled workers arose out of the United States' economic needs and resulted in giving immigration priority to persons with special skills judged to be in short supply in this country.

In essence, the 1965 Act modified the 1924 Immigration Act in the following two ways: 1) allowed unlimited immigration for spouses, unmarried children under the age of 21, and parents of U.S. citizens, and 2) increased the immigration quota for extended family members and people with special skills (Ong & Liu, 1994). Anticipating that there would be a greater number of immigration applicants than the allotted quota (20,000 immigrants from any one country with a cap of 120,000 and 170,000 for western and eastern hemispheres, respectively), the 1965 Act also established a preference system in which migrants meeting certain criteria had a higher likelihood of receiving a visa than other would be migrants. The lower number preference types were given higher priority for immigration.

1965 Immigration Act's Preference System

First Preference: Given to unmarried sons and daughters of U.S. citizens who are over the age of 21 years

Second Preference: Given to spouses and unmarried sons and daughters of aliens lawfully admitted for permanent residents

Third Preference: Given to members of the professionals or persons of exceptional ability in the science and arts

Fourth Preference: Given to married sons and daughters of U.S. citizens

| Fifth Preference: | Given to brothers and sisters of U.S. citizens who are more than 21 years old |
| Sixth Preference: | Given to skilled and unskilled workers in short supply |

Note: People who are spouses, unmarried children under the age of 21 years, or parents of U.S. citizens are not included in the preference system. They can enter as non-quota immigrants.

The groups that most benefited from the Immigration Act of 1965 were Asian Indians, Chinese, Filipinos, and South Koreans. As described in Chapter 1, approximately 1.9 million Asian Indians lived in the United States in 2000. Because only about 7,000 Asian Indians comprised the first arrivals in the early 1900s and no more Asian Indians were allowed until 1965, almost all of the Asian Indians living in the United States arrived as a result of the Immigration Act of 1965. Many of these immigrants, who entered the United States through the Third Preference, are from the middle and upper castes and from highly industrialized states such as Gujarat, Maharashtra, or Uttar Pradesh (Lessinger, 1995). A sizable number of these arrivals came not only with college degrees but also with postgraduate education or professional certification. For example, in 1980, 87.3 percent of New York State's recently arrived Asian Indians had completed high school and 60.8 percent four or more years of college (Lessinger, 1995). Recently, there also has been an increasing number of Asian Indians who have entered the United States through the other reunification-oriented preferences. Unlike their Third Preference counterparts, many of these individuals do not have high levels of education and unfortunately often work in low-paying jobs such as taxicab drivers and janitors.

As for Chinese Americans (including Taiwanese), there were nearly 2.9 million individuals living in the United States in 2000, comprising 24.2% of the Asian American population. This number represents a twelve-fold increase since 1960 when there were less than one-quarter of a million Chinese Americans. Chinese Americans immigrants came from a number of different countries including the People's Republic of China, Taiwan, Hong Kong, and Vietnam (many ethnic Chinese lived in Vietnam and left after the communist takeover in 1975; this group is described below). Like many other migrants, Chinese immigrants have come to the United States to seek better education for their children and long-term economic and political stability (Wong, 1998). Many Taiwanese immigrated to help their sons avoid the draft into the Taiwanese military (Uba, 1994). Many Chinese from Hong Kong immigrated because of the unknown future that laid ahead when Hong Kong was reverted to Chinese control in 1997. As for the immigrants from the People's Republic of China, they came to the United States to enjoy increased personal freedom and to be able to have more than one child per family (Wong, 1998). Many persons from the People's Republic of China also entered the United States as students and remained in the United States as political refugees; these persons are known as "status adjusters." For instance, when the Tiananmen Square massacre occurred in 1989, approximately 20,000 Chinese students studying in the United States were granted political asylum by the U.S. government.

As for the Filipino Americans, they number nearly 2.4 million persons and comprise the second largest Asian American group in the United States. In addition to the political, military, and cultural ties between the two countries that have existed since the United States colonized the Philippines in 1898, the lack of economic opportunities in the Philippines, especially for the well-educated Filipinas, served to make immigration to the United States an attractive option (Espiritu, 1995). Beginning in 1960, there became an overabundance of nurses, medical technicians, and pharmacists in the Philippines as a result of the U.S. investment in the education of Filipino health-related professionals to work for U.S. military during the war in Southeast Asia. When the United States withdrew in 1975, many female professionals could not find jobs that were comparable to their education levels. Fortunately for these individuals, there was a severe shortage of health professionals during that time in the United States and they were able to gain entrance.

South Korean immigrants represent another group that benefited from the 1965 Immigration Act. As of 2000, there were over 1.2 million Korean Americans living in the United States. The characteristics of South Korean emigrants between 1965 and early 1975 included the following: most were highly educated; most came through the Third Preference or the Sixth Preference; most came with some wealth; most came with families and were urban dwellers (from Seoul); and most were Christians (Yoon, 1997). Beginning in the late 1980s, there has been a decrease in the immigration of South Korean professionals, but an increase in white-collar workers (managerial, sales, and clerical occupations) and lower-class workers (manual laborers, farmers, and service workers) as a result of the increasing role of family networks as an entry mechanism (Yoon, 1997). The decrease in the number of immigrants who are professionals is the result of the fact that the professionals in South Korea during the 1980s have generally experienced an improvement in their socioeconomic status, thereby decreasing their desire to emigrate.

1975 TO THE PRESENT: THE LEGACY OF THE UNITED STATES' POLITICAL AND MILITARY INVOLVEMENT IN SOUTHEAST ASIA

Unlike the voluntary immigration of Asians as a result of the 1965 Immigration Act, the end of the U.S. involvement in the Vietnam War in 1975 created a very different motivation for migration of individuals from Southeast Asia. The U.S. involvement in Southeast Asia began in the mid-1950s as the French government withdrew from what was then known as French Indochina (areas covering Vietnam, Cambodia, and Laos) after the French forces were defeated in the First Indochina War (1946–1954). Immediately following the war, Laotians and Vietnamese were granted independence at the 1954 Geneva Conference (Chan, 1994). The Cambodians were granted independence the year before by the battle-weary French (Chan, 1994). However, for the Vietnamese, the newly found independence soon turned into a division of the country and to the establishment of North and South Vietnam. North Vietnam was aligned with the communist-bloc countries led by the then-Soviet Union, while South Vietnam aligned itself with capitalist countries led by the United States. During this period, the United States was in the midst of the Cold War as the U.S. foreign policy was dominated by the "domino theory" (Chan, 1994), which posited that if South Vietnam fell to Communism, the rest of Asia might fall in short order.

At first, the U.S. support for South Vietnam came in the form of weapons, advisors, and money as the South Vietnamese government tried to defend itself from the North Vietnamese who were beginning their efforts to unify the country (Chan, 1994). But by the mid-1970s, the U.S. involvement escalated to a full-scale war against the North Vietnamese Army (Rumbaut, 1995). The U.S. soldiers fought side-by-side with their South Vietnamese counterparts and U.S. bombers frequently struck North Vietnam. After discovering that the North Vietnamese were transporting weapons through a mountainous path, called the Ho Chi Minh Trail, located within the border of neighboring Laos, U.S. planes also began to conduct illegal bombing runs into Laotian territory; because the United States had not declared war with Laos or obtained permission from the Laotian government to drop bombs on its territory, these bombing runs were found to be illegal (Chan, 1994). In addition, the U.S. Central Intelligence Agency hired the Hmong, the people living in the mountains of Laos, to fight for the United States against the North Vietnamese forces as well as the Laotian communist group known as the Pathet Lao (Chan, 1994). However, despite these efforts, U.S. military leaders realized that it was impossible for the United States and the South Vietnamese forces to be victorious. Finally in April 1975, the United States withdrew its forces from South Vietnam and the rest of Southeast Asia. By this time, 2.2 million American soldiers had served in Vietnam and almost 58,000 had died there or were missing in action (Rumbaut, 1995).

The United States decision to leave Southeast Asia left many South Vietnamese people in a quandary (Freeman, 1994; Rumbaut, 1994). Thousands of South Vietnamese were connected to the United States through their military service or employment with the U.S. embassy (Freeman, 1994; Rumbaut, 1994). With the impending takeover by the Communist North Vietnamese forces, these people were afraid for their lives. By the end of April 1975, the U.S. military and government flew thousands of these people, mostly South Vietnamese military and government officials, to the United States (Freeman, 1994; Rumbaut, 1994). However, this effort only made a small dent in the total number of South Vietnamese who wished to leave the country. As a result, thousands of Vietnamese who had some connections with the United States, and thus were afraid for their lives, fled by foot to refugee camps in neighboring countries, mainly Thailand, and by boat to Hong Kong and as far south as Australia (Freeman, 1994; Rumbaut, 1994). Unfortunately, many of these people died during their voyage because their ships were not seaworthy (Freeman, 1994; Rumbaut, 1994).

The situation for the Hmong and Laotians who were connected with the U.S. government and military was no less grim. They also faced the possibility of persecution by the Laotian Communist forces, which also became victorious when the United States decided to pull out of Southeast Asia (Chan, 1994). As a result, these people fled Laos and sought safety in refugee camps in neighboring countries, mainly Thailand.

For the Cambodians, the situation was somewhat different (Etcheson, 1984). After the country gained its independence in 1953, Cambodia was ruled by Prince Sihanouk. However, similar to Vietnam and Laos, the Communist forces in Cambodia, called the Khmer Rouge, began to fight for control of the country. In 1975, the Khmer Rouge took control of Phnom Penh, the capital of Cambodia, and declared the formation of a new Cambodia, a society with no individuality, no property, no system of extended family, and no cultural heritage (Etcheson, 1984). The Khmer Rouge declared 1975 to be the Year Zero indicating the birth of this new society (Etcheson, 1984). However, the Khmer Rouge's plans exacted a heavy price on its people. First, in an attempt to eradicate the old Cambodia, the Khmer Rouge first executed most of Cambodia's educated people who were in the professional occupations and persons who worked for the government or the military (Etcheson, 1984). Anyone who wore glasses was killed because they were thought to be well educated. Phnom Penh was also evacuated and all of its residents were sent to the countryside to farm and make a new living, but many of these people starved to death because they were not given any farm tools or seeds (Etcheson, 1984). Until 1978, the year when the Vietnamese military forced the Khmer Rouge from power, at least 2 million Cambodians, or one-third of the entire population, died by the hands of the Khmer Rouge; some estimates are as high as one-half of the population (Etcheson, 1984). Fortunately others, however, were able to escape to Thailand and were eventually able to seek refuge in the United States.

Given these grave situations in Southeast Asia, the United States decided to allow most of these persons to enter the country. In 1975 alone, the United States allowed 125,000 Vietnamese refugees, 800 Laotian refugees, and 4,600 Cambodian refugees to enter the country (Rumbaut, 1995). The influx of refugees continued. The influx of refugees continued thereafter. A total of 653,521 Vietnamese refugees, 230,023 Laotian and Hmong refugees, and 147,460 Cambodian refugees entered the United States between 1975 and 1992 (Rumbaut, 1995). Also included among the Vietnamese refugees were ethnic Chinese who lived in Vietnam for decades but still identified themselves ethnically as Chinese (Freeman, 1995). In addition to these refugees, 173,896 Vietnamese entered the United States as immigrants after the passing of the 1989 Orderly Departure Program, a provision to prevent the dangerous outflow of refugees and allow Vietnamese to immigrate to the United States (Rumbaut, 1995).

Unfortunately, the refugees and subsequent immigrants from Southeast Asia have not fared well in the United States. Most did not speak English well and most had completed only high school education (Rumbaut, 1995). For example, one study of these refugees revealed that 66% professed no English proficiency at all, 20% indicated barest proficiency, 10% knew some English but not well, and the rest possessed a reasonable grasp of the language

(Caplan, Whitmore, & Choy, 1989). As a result, many of these individuals suffered from culture shock and difficulties in adjusting to their new lives in the United States. One area where these problems are visible is in the high percentage of Southeast Asians who live in poverty, as discussed in Chapter 1. In addition, many of these individuals suffer from the traumas of war and of being refugees. Hence, Southeast Asian Americans represent a significant challenge to mental health professionals in providing appropriate services.

SUMMARY AND CONCLUSIONS

In this chapter, I have described the varied immigration histories among Asian American ethnic groups. The histories range from the early arrivals in the mid-1800's to the current arrivals, and include various reasons for (e.g., voluntary vs. involuntary) and experiences after migration. However, one commonality that exists among all of the groups is that they and their descendants have had to adjust to many difficulties as members of a minority group in the United States. In fact, we saw that many Asian Americans were faced with outright prejudice and mistreatment by the rest of the society at many points in history. Nonetheless, Asian Americans have persevered and laid a strong foundation in the United States, and now represent a significant and visible segment of the American society.

For counselors to be effective with Asian American clients, they must be knowledgeable about these experiences, of trials and tribulations endured by Asian Americans throughout their history in the United States. In addition, counselors need to know about the current oppressions experienced by Asian Americans. In the next chapter, I will focus on this issue.

CHAPTER 3

Current Status of Asian Americans

Like other racial minority groups in the United States, Asian Americans have been and continue to be victims of racism, stereotyping, and other forms of oppression as a result of having different physical and sociocultural characteristics in comparison to the dominant European American group. In Chapter 2, I described some of the historical injustices experienced by Asian Americans, which ranged from racist immigration policies (e.g., 1882 Chinese Exclusion Act) to the internment of an entire Asian American ethnic group (Japanese Americans). In this chapter, I describe the present-day oppression faced by Asian Americans. Specifically, I focus on the areas of oppression that affect the mental health of Asian Americans, including racism, stereotyping, the model minority myth, acculturative stress, and occupational problems. Also, I discuss intergenerational conflict, which is an area of mental health that is particularly relevant to Asian American families. Then, I conclude the chapter by describing various sources of strengths and resiliency among Asian Americans that have served as strong buffers against these mental health risk factors. As you read this chapter, please consider the following questions.

- *What types of oppression are Asian Americans currently experiencing?*

- *How are these experiences of oppression related to those of the past?*

- *How do the current experiences of oppression compare in terms of type and magnitude to those experiences of the past?*

- *How might current oppression affect the psychological functioning of Asian Americans?*

- What are the sources of resilience used among Asian Americans to deal with the oppression they face?

- What are your personal thoughts and feelings about Asian Americans?

- What stereotypes and prejudices about Asian Americans do you have?

- How might these attitudes affect your work with Asian American clients?

RACISM

The Fresno Bee, a newspaper in Fresno, California, published an article containing the following report:

> Vandals spray-painted racist graffiti on the Gurdwara Sahib temple in Fresno over the weekend. Evidence of the crime remained Sunday as Sikhs gathered for services. Two large blue scrawls in front of the Sikh Association of Fresno temple warned: "Rags Go Home" and "It's Not Your Country." Another message—this one with a religious/cultural slur and a four-letter obscenity—was scribbled on a rear door.

The above caption from a newspaper article was published not in the early 1900s when such acts were condoned and even encouraged, but on March 15, 2004. Despite some of the advances the United States has made during the Civil Rights Movement of the 1960s, racism in the United States, in general and specifically toward Asian Americans, is still a far too common occurrence. Racism involves "the subordination of members of targeted racial groups who have relatively little social power (i.e. Blacks, Latino/as, Native Americans and Asians), by members of the agent racial group who have relatively more power (i.e. Whites)" (Wijeyesinghe, Griffin, & Love, 1997, p. 88). Racism can be either active or passive and can occur at various levels, including institutional (e.g., discriminatory laws), societal (e.g., race hate-groups), and individual (e.g., racial slurs by an individual). As I described in Chapter 2, the history of the United States is fraught with racist actions against Asian Americans (Chan, 2001). In recent years, there has been an increase in reports of anti-Asian vandalism, intimidation and threats, and incidents involving bodily harm (National Asian Pacific Legal Consortium, 1999, 2002). For instance, between 1998 and 1999, incidents involving aggravated assault increased by 23% and threats and intimidation increased by 34%. In their most recent report, the National Asian Pacific Legal Consortium (2002) reported that there were nearly 250 incidents against Asian Americans, particularly South Asians, in the three months immediately following the terrorist attacks of September 11, 2001. Also, a survey of over 1,200 adults by the Committee of 100 (2001) found that about 25% would feel uncomfortable having an Asian American as president of the United States, whereas 15% felt the same way for an African American and 14% for a woman. About half of the respondents believed that Chinese Americans would be more loyal to China than to the United States. About 25% reported that they would feel uncomfortable if someone in their family married an Asian American. Nearly 20% reported that they would feel upset if large numbers of Asian Americans moved into their neighborhoods.

Despite the prevalence of racism toward Asian Americans, there has been a lack of attention on this phenomenon (Hune & Chan, 1997). Several scholars (Espiritu, 1997; Hune & Chan, 1997; Young & Takeuchi, 1998) have explained that this inattention may be the result of the tendency of Americans to dichotomize racial issues in terms of a two-tiered racial order, with whites at one end and Blacks at the other end. Espiritu (1997) noted that Asian Americans are considered neither Black nor white, but at the same time either Black or white. This statement implies that Asian Americans are sometimes considered a part of the dominant group and other times a part of a minority group, but rarely a group of its own. As a result, the experiences of Asian Americans regarding racism are often overlooked and overshadowed by the experiences of whites and Blacks.

There have been a number of empirical studies that have examined the relationship between racist events and mental health status (e.g., Fischer & Shaw, 1999), although they typically have not included the experiences of Asian Americans and were largely based on data from African American participants. In general, these studies suggest a positive relationship between racism and physiological stress (e.g., Fang & Myers, 2001) and an inverse relationship between racism and both life satisfaction and self-esteem (e.g., Broman, 1997). Specific to Asian Americans, I was able to find only one empirical study. Asamen and Berry (1987) reported a significant negative correlation between perceived prejudice and self-concept among Japanese Americans. Nonetheless, even without much empirical evidence, it is reasonable to assume that a racist event can have serious deleterious affects on the mental health of Asian Americans.

Liang, Li, and Kim (2004) published an instrument to measure the racism-related stress experienced by Asian Americans. Named the *Asian American Racism-Related Stress Inventory* (AARRSI), this instrument allows respondents to indicate the degree to which they felt upset when they experienced various types of racist events. The events described in the instrument have been categorized across three domains: socio-historical, perpetual foreigner, and general. For the socio-historical domain, examples of racist incidents include: "You learn that most non-Asian Americans are ignorant of the oppression and racial prejudice Asian Americans have endured in the United States," "You notice that U.S. history books offer no information of the contributions of Asian Americans," and "You hear about a racially motivated murder of an Asian American man." Examples of incidents in the perpetual domain include: "You are told that 'you speak English so well,'" "You are asked where you are really from," and "Someone asks you what your real name is." For the general domain, examples of incidents include: "A student you don't know asks you for help in math," "Someone assumes that they serve dog meat in Asian restaurants," and "Someone asks you if you can teach him/her karate." It is hoped that the availability of this instrument will encourage further research in the area of racism-related stress among Asian Americans. Also, counselors might perhaps consider using this instrument to assess their

Asian American clients' experiences with racism and the related stress. At a minimum, the items in the instrument could give counselors a starting point to discussing the kinds of oppression experienced by their clients.

Recently, the attention to racism has been in the form of what is known as racial microaggressions (Sue et al., 2007). Sue et al. (2007) defined racial microaggressions as "brief and commonplace daily verbal, behavioral, or environmental indignities, whether intentional or unintentional, that communicate hostile, derogatory, or negative racial slights and insults toward people of color." It is believed that people who commit these racial microaggressions are often unaware that they are engaging in this type of offense when they interact with racial minorities, including Asian Americans. Although research is just emerging on this topic, examples cited by Sue et al. include assuming Asian Americans to be foreign-born ("Where are you from?"), ascribing intelligence based on race (assuming Asian Americans are good in math), and pathologizing cultural values (assuming a quiet Asian American as not capable of being a good leader).

STEREOTYPING

Stereotypes refer to a set of traits believed to be characteristic of a social category (Greenwald & Banaji, 1995). In functional terms, when an individual is perceived as being a member of a particular stereotyped group, the group-relevant cognitive structure is activated, and subsequent applications of this information (such as judgments and attitudes) are processed within the framework of that particular stereotype. For example:

- When someone says, "That woman is an Asian American," what stereotypes does this statement raise for you? How about quiet, timid, and unassertive? Or perhaps exotic, sexual, and accommodating?
- What about when someone says, "That man is an Asian American?" what stereotypes does this statement raise for you? Perhaps nerd, asexual, kung fu master, and hypermasculine?

Stereotypes of Asian Americans have evolved over the years. Initially, stereotypes of Chinese migrants in the 1850s were neutral when they were viewed as a useful labor source: yellow skinned, slant eyed, and pigtailed. But, the stereotypes became negative as they came into direct job competition with European Americans. Soon, Chinese workers were associated with inherent qualities: filthy, immoral, treacherous, unintelligent, cowardly, and incapable of assimilation. Similarly, stereotypes of Japanese migrants were subject to transformation. Initially, Japanese laborers were seen as industrious, hardworking, and wise. However, as they came into competition for jobs, the stereotypes of Chinese not only quickly generalized to Japanese but they became more severe. Japanese laborers were viewed as immoral, sneaky, and sexually aggressive. These stereotypes were further intensified when the Japanese attacked Pearl Harbor in 1941. Many Americans viewed Japanese Americans as perpetual foreigners (e.g., "Jap is Jap" regardless of birthplace) and perceived them as deceitful, cruel, vicious, and two-faced.

More recently, the stereotypes about Asian Americans have taken a dual characteristic. Asian men have been portrayed as hypermasculine (e.g., a martial artist) or effeminate (e.g., a studious nerd). Asian women have been portrayed as superfeminine (e.g., the image of the geisha girl) or castrating (e.g., the image of the "Dragon Lady") (Espiritu, 1997). Asian Americans also have been considered diligent, intelligent, law abiding, industrious, quiet and shy, frugal, and willing to sacrifice the present for the future. In addition, they have been portrayed as good students, skilled in math, do not cheat, timid, quiet, speech anxious, shy, conforming, competitive, reserved, hardworking, thrifty, and perpetual foreigners. So, are all of these stereotypes bad? How about the positive ones?

While it may seem that some of the stereotypes shed seemingly positive light on Asian Americans, "positive" stereotypes may conflict with or serve to emphasize the stereotypes of the larger society (Sue & Sue, 2003). For example, the Asian American male stereotype of being quiet conflicts with the accepted sex role stereotype of the U.S. culture. The Asian American female stereotype of being conforming perpetuates sexism and eroticism. "Positive" stereotypes also tend to overlook problems such as the lack of parity in salary per educational attainment, the glass ceiling effect, poverty in the ghettos, and gang warfare. Furthermore, and perhaps most importantly, all stereotypes overlook the uniqueness of Asian American individuals.

MODEL MINORITY MYTH

Karen is a 45-year-old first-generation Laotian American woman who works as a sales clerk at a local grocery store. She has been married for 20 years and has two teenagers. After arriving in the United States as a refugee in 1975 at the age 14 years, Karen has had a lot of difficulties adjusting to her new life in this country. Due to the language difficulty and her family's financial problems, Karen was forced to drop out of high school to work and help support her family. Without a high school diploma, Karen has been stuck at the lowest end of the pay scale at her position. Karen's husband, who also entered the United States as a refugee in 1975, has not fared well either. Although he has a high school diploma, he has not had a permanent job for the past 10 years. Because he has no specialized training, Karen's husband has had to move from one temporary job to another, mostly as a site laborer for construction companies. For some time now, Karen's husband has been drinking heavily as a way to pass the time between jobs. Karen suspects that her husband also might be suffering from severe depression. One day at work, Karen speaks to a co-worker who complains about the difficulties she is having at home. At one point, the co-worker states, "You are so lucky to be an Asian, Karen. Asian Americans always seem to be doing well and never have any problems."

One stereotype that has long-affected Asian Americans is that of the "model minority." First coined by sociologist William Peterson (1966), the notion of model minority suggests that Asian Americans embody the modern day American success story. That is, Asian Americans are functioning well in society, are somehow immune from cultural conflicts and discrimination, and experience few adjustment difficulties. Hune and Chan (1997) explained that the model minority myth has resulted in the perception of Asian Americans as be-ing "well-behaved, diligent high achievers who persevere and are educationally successful despite socioeconomic and linguistic obstacles" (p. 44). Furthermore, as a model minority, all Asian Americans are viewed as diligent, frugal, and willing to sacrifice the present for the future, a set of characteristics that some believe has helped Asian Americans gain upward mobility and public accolades (Crystal, 1989).

Sue (1994) notes that the model minority myth has masked the real social and economic problems encountered by large segments of the Asian American population and diverted attention away from the discrimination and prejudice that affect their lives. In addition, applying the model minority myth to all Asian Americans has helped to downplay existing within-group differences. Furthermore, the model minority myth has often fostered or created hostile feelings between Asian Americans and other racial minority groups. Sue's points are further delineated by Crystal (1989), who notes that the model minority myth has

> obscured many serious problems in the Asian community and has been used to justify omitting Asian Americans from federal funding and some special minority programs. Moreover, the Asian-American success story has been turned into a weapon against other minorities by persons who deny the existence of racism in America. (p. 405)

Kim (1973) also pointed out that the model minority myth has excluded Asian Americans from receiving attention relative to education, health, hous-ing, employment, social welfare programs, and economic opportunities.

Proponents of the model minority myth point to four major findings in support of their contention: (1) higher than average earnings; (2) educational success; and (3) positive indications of mental health. It is true that the Asian American median family income is higher than the rest of the U.S. population (Reeves & Bennett, 2003). However, Asian American families consist of more members than European American families, which suggests that there are more income earners in Asian American families (Reeves & Bennett, 2003). Consistent with this point, the median per capita income for Asian Americans was reported to be $29,901, whereas for European Americans it was $31,051 (DeNavas-Walt et al., 2008). Also, for Asian Americans (and Pacific Islanders) over 25 years old and with a bachelor's degree or more, their median per ca-pita income was $41,370 for men and $32,450 for women, in comparison to $50,240 for European American men and $34,250 for European American women (U.S. Bureau of the Census, 1997). Here, a clear disparity can be seen on income level across the same level of educational attainment. In addition, a strong disparity between men and women for both groups also can be clearly seen. Moreover, although the rate of impoverishment among Asian Americans as a group is lower than the national average, the incidence of poverty among Asian Americans was 20% higher than that of European Americans (Reeves & Bennett, 2003).

Statistics also indicate a significant within-group difference among Asian Americans relative to income. In 1995, the median family income levels for Vietnamese Americans, Laotian Americans, Hmong Americans, and Cambodian

TABLE **1**
Demographic Characteristics of Southeast Asian Americans

Median Family Income in 1995				
Cambodian	Hmong	Laotian	Vietnamese	U.S. Average
$18,126	$14,327	$23,101	$30,550	$35,225
Poverty Rate in 1995				
Cambodian	Hmong	Laotian	Vietnamese	U.S. Average
42.6%	63.6%	25.7%	25.7%	13.1%

Americans were far below the national average (see Table 1; Rumbaut, 1995). Also, the poverty rates among Cambodian Americans, Vietnamese Americans, Laotian Americans, and Hmong Americans were much higher than the national average (see Table 1; Rumbaut, 1995).

In terms of Asian Americans' higher educational attainment, it is true that on average, Asian Americans have a higher rate of achieving a bachelors or an advanced degree than European Americans (Bauman & Graf, 2003). However, Reeves and Bennett (2003) found that Asians (and Pacific Islanders) were almost twice as likely to have less than a ninth-grade education as European Americans. Furthermore, in 1990, the percentages of Hmong American, Laotian American, Cambodian American, and Vietnamese American individuals with bachelor's degrees or greater were only 2.2, 4.6, 4.8, and 12.4, respectively, whereas the averages for European Americans, Japanese Americans, and Chinese Americans were 25.0 percent, 24.4 percent, and 21.7 percent, respectively. Also, as mentioned above, Asian Americans tend to receive lower pay in comparison to other Americans with comparable educational attainment (U.S. Bureau of the Census, 1997).

It is true that Asian Americans have lower rates of utilization of mental health services in comparison to other Americans (Snowden & Cheung, 1990). However, the lower rates do not necessarily indicate a population free from psychological problems. Mental health researchers now believe that underutilization of mental health services by Asian Americans is related to cultural factors such as loyalty to family, sensitivity to shame, preference for indigenous healers, and the mismatch between the cultural values among Asian Americans and the values inherent in Western mental health services (Atkinson, 2004).

ACCULTURATIVE STRESS

Imagine that you have moved to another country where the language and culture are very different from those of the United States.

- What difficulties might you face as soon as you arrive in this country?
- How would you go about finding a place to live and buying groceries?
- How would you cope with the language and cultural differences?

- What kinds of psychological effects would living in this foreign land have on you?

Despite the various migration histories and social, political, and economic experiences of Asian Americans, one experience that is shared by all Asian Americans is acculturation to the dominant U.S. culture. According to Graves (1967), acculturation refers to the changes in behavior, values, identity, and attitudes that an individual experiences as a result of being in contact with other cultures. For example, changes occur as an acculturating individual acquires a new language, religion, modes of dress, schooling, transportation, housing, and forms of social organization and social relations with the dominant group.

Berry and Annis (1974) noted that members of immigrant ethnic minority groups, including Asian Americans, are vulnerable to stresses arising out of the acculturation process, and have labeled this phenomenon "acculturative stress." More formally, Nwadiora and McAdoo (1996) defined acculturative stress as "Psychocultural stress due to cultural differences found between a host culture and an incoming culture marked by reduction in the physical and mental health status of individuals or groups undergoing acculturation" (p. 477). For Asian Americans, the extent to which they experience acculturative stress is moderated by factors such as their immigration history and related socioeconomic status. For example, it can be expected that a third-generation Chinese American son of a physician could be expected to suffer less acculturative stress than a first-generation Laotian refugee.

Psychological symptoms of acculturative stress include lowered mental health status (e.g., confusion, anxiety, depression), feelings of marginality and alienation, heightened psychosomatic symptom level and identity confusion (Berry & Annis, 1974). Acculturative stress has the following effects on one's life: ineffective decision making process, impairment of occupational functioning, contribution to role entrapment, status leveling, heightened emotional strain, and possible contribution to ineffective client-counselor relations (Smart & Smart, 1995). Smart and Smart explained that people with acculturative stress tend to narrow the range of options that they perceive as viable. These people have decreased abilities to make decisions with clarity and resolution and to carry them out effectively. Acculturative stress impairs occupational functioning because psychosocial functioning is closely related to vocational functioning. Acculturative stress also causes Asian Americans to experience heightened emotional stress and feelings of hopelessness. They may acquiesce to such feelings as "things will be better for the next generation" and "my job success was not meant to be." A meta-analytic study by Moyerman and Forman (1992) that included an analysis of 49 studies of acculturation and adjustment found that stress and anxiety among Asian Americans may be acute at the very beginning of the acculturation process, but gradually becomes less pronounced. These authors also found that acculturative stress is positively correlated with psychosocial and health problems. In a study on the effects of negative life events such as acculturative stress, Rabkin and Streuning (1976) found that "life events may account for at least 9 percent of the variance in illness" (p. 1015). Other studies have also found correlations between acculturative stress and depression among Asian Americans (Nicassio, Solomon, Guest, & McCullough, 1986; Shin, 1994). Acknowledging the significance of this phenomenon, the *Diagnostic and Statistical Manual of Mental Disorders* (American Psychiatric Association, 1994) has given a diagnostic label (V62.4 Acculturation Problem) to the problems associated with acculturation. In the counseling context, acculturative stress may contribute to strained and ineffective client-counselor relationships and decreased therapeutic alliance.

INTERGENERATIONAL CONFLICT

Similar to individuals who experience acculturative stress, Asian American families as a whole also may experience adjustment difficulties. One of these difficulties is intergenerational conflict, which may occur when family members acculturate at different rates. For example, consider a Pakistani American adolescent who immigrated two years ago and has been attending a local middle school. It is possible that this individual will acculturate at a faster rate than her parents because she is constantly exposed to the dominant U.S. culture at her school. Due to the strong environmental influences that exist in the school, this student could begin to adhere more strongly to dominant U.S. cultural norms than her parents while at the same time lose some of her Pakistani cultural norms. Consequently, this situation could create problems between the adolescent and parents, due to the varying value system that has developed.

Consistent with this idea, Hwang (2007) used the term Acculturative Family Distancing (AFD) to describe the family functioning among Asian Americans with respect to varying levels of adaptation by parents and children to the dominant U.S. and traditional Asian cultural norms. Specifically, AFD is described as "the problematic distancing that occurs between immigrant parents and children that is a consequence of differences in acculturative [and enculturative] processes and cultural changes that become more salient over time" (p. 398). Hwang posited that AFD increases the development of problems through distancing in the realms of emotion, cognition, and behavior, which eventually lead to family conflict.

In support of this model, Chung (2001) documented the presence of intergenerational conflicts among Asian American college students in California. In one of the first studies on this topic with Asian Americans, Chung assessed intergenerational conflict across three dimensions: family expectations, education and career, and dating and marriage. Some of the areas of intergenerational conflicts for the family expectations dimension include: lack of communication with parents, following cultural traditions, pressure to learn one's own Asian language, expectations based on being male or female, and expectations based on birth order. Some of the areas of intergenerational conflicts for the education and career dimension include: how much time to spend on studying, recreation, sports, and practicing music; importance of academic achievement; emphasis on materialism and success; which school to attend and which major to study; and which career to pursue. For the dating and marriage dimension, areas of intergenerational conflict include: when to begin dating, whom to date, and whom to marry. In Chung's study, the respondents were asked to indicate the extent to which each of these areas was a source of conflict between them and their parents.

Based on data from 342 students, Chung (2001) found that male Asian American students reported less conflict on dating and marriage than their female counterparts. In addition, Japanese American students reported less conflict in this area than Chinese, Filipino, Korean, and Southeast Asian Americans. For the dimension of family expectations, Japanese American students reported less intergenerational conflict than Korean and Southeast Asian Americans. Also, for this dimension and the dimension of education and career, a group that was classified as being highly acculturated had lower conflict than two groups that were deemed to be either minimally acculturated or bicultural. In sum, this study presents an interesting picture on the presence and type of intergenerational conflict among Asian Americans. However, more research is needed to study this phenomenon, particularly as it is related to mental health outcome. Also, given the continued influx of Asian immigrants to the United States, it will be important to examine this topic further.

In terms of studies directly examining the relation between the intergenerational gap along cultural values (cultural values gap) and parent-child conflict, Ahn, Kim, and Park (2008) found that as the Asian cultural values gap increased between Korean American parents and their children, the family experienced greater intensity of conflicts, particularly in the area of dating and marriage. Interestingly, Ahn et al.'s study revealed that as one's ability to be cognitively flexible increased the intensity of conflicts in the area of dating and marriage decreased. However, as the Korean American children use of the social support coping strategy increased, so did the intensity of conflicts. In a study that examined Asian Americans as a whole, Tsai-Chae and Nagata (2008) also found that as the cultural values gap increased between parents and children, so did the extent of parent-child conflicts. These studies provide initial information on the type and extent of difficulties that are experienced by Asian Americans parents and children as their cultural norms diverge.

OCCUPATIONAL PROBLEMS

Asian Americans, both foreign-born and U.S.-born, have experienced a number of occupational problems that place them at risk for psychological problems. While many of the recently arrived Asian immigrants entered the United States for various social and political reasons, a majority of these persons migrated to the United States for economic reasons; that is, with a desire for more secure and rewarding economic opportunities and upward socioeconomic mobility (Ong, Bonacich, & Cheng, 1994). However, observations of their vocational behaviors suggest that these immigrants' career aspirations and expectations have not been met (Min, 1996).

As I described in Chapter 2, the Immigration Act of 1965 established a preferential system of visa distribution favoring family reunification and the immigration of highly educated professionals. As a result of this criterion, a large number of doctors, nurses, pharmacists, and scientists immigrated to the United States, particularly in the years just subsequent to 1965. While many of these persons were able to find occupational positions that were comparable to their education levels, a majority of them were forced to settle for positions that were less than comparable due to cultural and language difficulties (Kim, 1981; Lessinger, 1995; Ong, Bonacich, & Cheng, 1994; Yoon, 1993). For example, sociological studies of Asian Indian, Filipino, and South Korean immigrants found that, despite their medical or nursing degrees from prestigious universities, these persons tended to obtain positions in second- or third-rate hospitals, were forced to choose low-paying fringe specialties, and entered into occupations in fields other than their areas of specialization (Kim, 1981; Lessinger, 1995; Ong et al., 1994; Yoon, 1993). Also, foreign-trained Filipino nurses have been forced into positions such as a nurse-aide and other positions for which they are overqualified (Ong et al., 1994). Other studies have also found that many graduate-level educated immigrants, particularly Koreans, are forced to go into small businesses (e.g., liquor stores, fruit and vegetable stands, small grocery stores) because they are not able to obtain jobs whose salaries and position statuses are comparable to their educational levels (Min, 1996; Lessinger, 1995; Ong et al., 1994). Based on these findings, Kincaid and Yum (1987) concluded that many Asian Americans have experienced a significant drop in occupational prestige and the concomitant downward economic mobility.

Unfortunately, U.S.-born Asian Americans are not faring any better in their vocational endeavors. As described above, at the same levels of educational attainment, there is a significant disparity on income level between Asian Americans and European Americans (U.S. Bureau of the Census, 1997). Also, Asian Americans tend to work in a narrow group of occupations (Leong & Serafica, 1995). They tend to be overrepresented in medicine, biological and life sciences, engineering, architecture, and accounting, but underrepresented in the fields of law, politics, sports, arts, and entertainment (Leong & Serafica, 1995). These findings may suggest that Asian Americans tend to have a restricted range of occupational interests and may view the barriers for the occupations in these underrepresented areas as too difficult to overcome. They also may suggest that Asian Americans could be stereotyped as having abilities for only certain types of occupations but not others and are not encouraged to enter the areas in which they are underrepresented.

Given this situation, it is possible that U.S.-born Asian Americans may endure greater psychological suffering from limited job opportunities than recently immigrated Asian Americans. Because the U.S.-born Asian Americans may have preconceived expectations of equal opportunities by the virtue of their birth in the United States, they may not be resilient to facing limited employment opportunities and experiencing job discrimination. In other words, while foreign-born Asian Americans may enter the United States with expectations of vocational difficulties including racial discrimination, the U.S.-born Asian Americans may not have such buffering expectations and thus be unprepared to effectively cope with occupational mistreatment. As a result, U.S.-born Asian Americans may be negatively impacted by racism and discrimination with even greater psychological intensity than recently immigrated Asian Americans.

The Los Angeles Riots of 1992

The three-day riot that occurred in Los Angeles in 1992 illustrates one of the problems that may be related to the narrow range of occupational options available to Asian Americans. As mentioned above, Korean Americans have tended to establish small businesses because they are not able to obtain jobs whose salaries and position status were comparable to their educational levels. As such, there was an overrepresentation of Korean Americans operating small businesses in South Central Los Angeles, the site of the tragic event.

The Los Angeles Riots (also known as the Civil Unrest of Los Angeles) began on April 29, 1992, after four white officers from the Los Angeles Police Department were acquitted on charges of using excessive force against Rodney King, a 25-year old black motorist who was beaten by the police when he refused to comply with their order to surrender. The beating was caught on videotape and shown repeatedly as evidence of police brutality against African Americans. Immediately following the verdict, areas surrounding South Central Los Angeles became focal points of protest by African Americans. However, these protests soon turned violent and many businesses in these areas were vandalized, looted, and destroyed. Of the total of 4,500 stores that were either burned down or looted, 2,300 were Korean-owned, and of the total of $1 billion in property damages, $400 million were borne by Korean Americans (Yoon, 1997).

There has been much discussion about the reasons why Korean American merchants suffered disproportionate amounts of damage (e.g., Min, 1996; Yoon, 1997). Min (1996) offered several possible reasons, one of which was based on the middleman minority and scapegoating theories. According to the these theories, inner-city African Americans were frustrated at being unable to improve their economic condition in South Central Los Angeles and vented their frustrations and aggression on their nearest and most convenient target, the Korean American merchants. Min also explained that the media might have contributed to the riots by repeatedly showing a videotape of a Korean American merchant shooting an African American girl who the merchant believed was robbing the store, and then the videotape of King being beaten by the police, thereby equating the two incidents. The pairing of these videos may have further galvanized African Americans' anger toward the Los Angeles Police Department, which then became directed toward Korean Americans. Also, Min pointed out that many African Americans believed that Korean American merchants exploited the African American communities by making profits, particularly through liquor stores, and not giving anything back to the communities in return. Lastly, Min noted that it is possible that Korean American merchants may have held negative stereotypes about African Americans, which may have led to rude behavior towards them. Whatever are the true reasons for the Los Angeles Riots, it is clear that the incident will represent one of the darkest periods of Korean American history in the United States.

RESILIENCY AND STRENGTHS

Positive Racial and Ethnic Identity

Despite the many difficulties faced by Asian Americans, it is also important to point out that Asian Americans have many strengths and high resiliency. One of the areas of strength and resiliency is positive racial and ethnic identity. There is evidence to suggest that many Asian Americans are proud of their racial and ethnic heritage. For example, based on qualitative interviews with Asian American college students, Kim, Brenner, Liang, and Asay (2003) found that many of the interviewees reported feeling very strongly connected with their culture of origin. According to these authors, a Filipino American male described, "I still act as a true Filipino, very humble and always respecting family and elders" (p. 164). An Asian Indian woman reported being open to her Indian culture and traditions and that she has "come to realize that India is the place for me" (p. 164). Similarly, a Korean American male explained, "I have a bigger desire for my Korean culture ... I'm more interested in listening to Korean music and watching Korean shows and dramas" (pp. 164–165). This finding is even more striking when considering that the interviewees were part of the 1.5-generation group (i.e., immigrated to the United States during adolescence), who presumably would have been exposed to the dominant U.S. culture to a greater extent than their immigrant parents.

In terms of other generations of Asian Americans and their positive racial and ethnic identity, Wei (1993) provides an illuminating description of how Asian Americans of varying ethnic groups, many of whom were descendants of immigrants from the late 1800s and early 1900s, were able to establish a positive Asian American identity during the Civil Rights Movement in the 1960s. During this period, Asian Americans were able to reclaim their racial and ethnic backgrounds and transform the perception of these backgrounds from being one of denial and embarrassment to one of pride and full embracement. As a result of these efforts, the present Asian American identity stands strong and continues to serve as a buffer against oppression experienced by Asian Americans.

The Community

An important source of the positive identity held by many Asian Americans is the presence of ethnic enclaves. Examples of these enclaves are the Chinatowns in San Francisco, Los Angeles, and New York City, Koreatown and Japantown in Los Angeles, Little Saigon in Westminster (CA), and Little India in New York City. These are the areas where one can find food, clothing, furniture, and other cultural artifacts related to the various ethnic groups. These also are the areas where individuals from these ethnic backgrounds can meet and interact with other people of the same background. To illustrate, the following is a description of Little India in New York City by Lessinger (1995):

> Virtually all of what is sold on 74th Street [Little India] is symbolic of Indian-ness, things largely first-generation immigrants feel, embody, and sum up a cultural identity of which they are very proud ... ethnic identity is both actively created and publicly demonstrated. Consumption is part of that process. Like other comparable immigrant shopping enclaves, Little India exists to provide the kinds

of things—at once utilitarian and badges of ethnicity—which immigrants cannot find in their own neighborhoods or local shopping malls. (p. 30)

The presence of these ethnic enclaves serves as an important source of cultural reinforcement and psychological resiliency against oppression. Asian Americans can visit their ethnic enclave to reconnect to and maintain their cultural histories, languages, traditions, and customs. In addition, the vibrant economic activities in many of these enclaves also can allow the Asian American ethnic community groups to facilitate cultural festivities, which further reinforce a positive cultural identity.

The Family

For Asian Americans, one of the most important cultural values is the sense of collectivism with immediate and extended families (see Kim, Atkinson, & Umemoto, 2001). Many Asian Americans view the family as the most important collective unit to which they belong. They will strive to bring honor to their families and maintain the family's well-being. They will avoid at all costs bringing shame and embarrassment to the family. In addition, Asian Americans will honor their parents and elders with respect, honor, fidelity, and devotion. They also will work to ensure that their siblings are cared for. Given the centrality of the family among Asian Americans, it is no wonder that the family serves as an important source of strength and resiliency. When Asian Americans face difficulties, they will turn to their family members first before turning to outside resources (Kim et al., 2003). They will look to the family to provide the necessary emotional support to overcome any difficulties. Hence, the family serves as an important buffer against discrimination and oppression experienced by Asian Americans.

The Cultural System

An additional source of psychological support for Asian Americans is the cultural system from which they have been socialized. The cultural system can be likened to a blueprint from which people's worldviews and meanings of psychological health are developed and manifested. To the extent that Asian Americans adhere to the beliefs and values of the Asian American cultural system, it can be anticipated that this form of congruence will lead to psychological health. In contrast, to the extent that Asian Americans do not adhere to the cultural system of their group, psychological problems can emerge. In terms of research bearing on this issue, studies have found that Asian American college students who adhere to Asian cultural values and behaviors tend to have more private-, membership-, and identity-related collective self-esteem (Kim & Omizo, 2005; Kim & Omizo, 2006). Similar findings were observed with Asian American high school students (Omizo, Kim, & Abel, 2008; Kim & Omizo, 2009). These findings suggest that Asian Americans who have a strong Asian value orientation tend to feel good about their Asian American group, believe that they are worthy members of the group, and perceive that their identity as an Asian American is an important part of their self-concept. In this way, the Asian American cultural system serves as an important source of strength and resiliency for many Asian Americans.

SUMMARY AND CONCLUSIONS

This chapter focuses on various risk factors faced by Asian Americans that can threaten their mental health. These risk factors include racism, stereotyping, the model minority myth, acculturative stress, intergenerational conflict, and occupational problems. Effectively dealing with these issues could present a significant challenge for counselors. First, counselors must become sensitive to the fact that these issues indeed are present in the lives of Asian Americans. Counselors also must become familiar with how these factors negatively affect Asian Americans' psychological functioning.

Second, counselors must become aware of their own thoughts and attitudes regarding these issues. For example, what are some of the racist and stereotyped thoughts you have about Asian Americans? What is your view about the model minority myth? How much have you bought into it? Also, what is the level of your acceptance of the fact that acculturative stress, intergenerational conflict, and occupational problems play significant roles in the lives of Asian Americans? For these questions, it is not so important to have the politically correct "positive responses." Rather, it is more important to think about them deeply and honestly for yourself so that you can raise the level of awareness about your own biases and prejudices.

Third, counselors need to think about what they can do to combat the oppressive conditions caused by racism, stereotyping, and the model minority myth, and consider how they might address these issues in their work with Asian American clients. Similarly, counselors need to think about how the issues of acculturative stress, intergenerational conflict, and occupational problems can be appropriately addressed in counseling. Perhaps a first step counselors can take to deal with these issues is to explore with their clients the degree to which these risk factors are present in the clients' lives and the extent to which the factors are related to the clients' presenting problems.

This chapter also focused on the areas of resiliency and strength among Asian Americans, specifically their positive racial and ethnic identity and the community, family, and cultural system as important sources of psychological support. Given these positive factors as potential buffers to psychological problems, it may be helpful for counselors to explore with their Asian American clients the extent to which these sources of strength and resilience are present in the clients' lives and how they can be further cultivated. Now, let's turn our attention to a more in depth exploration about the Asian American cultural system.

CHAPTER 4

Asian American Cultural Systems

Effective counseling with Asian American clients requires a thorough understanding of the cultural systems in which they have been socialized. Because there is a high degree of diversity among Asian Americans, particularly as they relate to the varied ethnic backgrounds and immigration histories, gaining a good understanding of Asian Americans' experiences requires a conceptual framework that can help discern this within-group diversity. The theories of acculturation and enculturation and racial/ethnic identity development can be very helpful in this regard. Therefore, in this section, I describe these adaptation theories as they relate to Asian Americans. In addition, I present cultural values that are salient to Asian Americans, as well as important similarities and differences among various Asian ethnic groups on their adherence to these values. The focus on cultural values is based on the idea that these values have important implications for counseling Asian Americans. As you read this chapter, please consider the following questions.

- What conceptual frameworks presented here are helpful for you to understand the within-group diversity among Asian Americans?

- What are the cultural values that are salient to Asian Americans?

- How are these values similar or dissimilar to your own cultural values?

- If these values are similar or different from your own values, what implications do they have for you when counseling Asian Americans?

A THEORY OF ACCULTURATION AND ENCULTURATION

As described in the previous chapters, Asian Americans comprise individuals with diverse migration histories. Many individuals are five and six generations removed from their ancestors who migrated to the United States between the mid-1800s and early 1900s. Others are third- and fourth-generation Americans whose ancestors entered the United States during World War II and the Korean War. There are also Asian Americans who entered after the passing of the Immigration Act of 1965 or after the United States pulled out of Southeast Asia, as well as their second- and third-generation children. Furthermore, Asian Americans can comprise individuals who arrived from an Asian country just yesterday. This diversity with respect to length of residence indicates that Asian Americans represent a dramatic range in the degree to which they have adapted to the norms of the dominant U.S. culture, and to which they have retained the norms of the Asian culture. To understand this type of diversity that is related to differential levels of adaptation, the theory of acculturation and enculturation can be helpful.

Acculturation was first defined by Redfield, Linton, and Herskovits (1936) as follows: "Acculturation comprehends those phenomena which result when groups of individuals sharing different cultures come into continuous first-hand contact, with subsequent changes in the original culture patterns of either or both groups" (pp. 149-152). Three decades later, Graves (1967) coined the term *psychological acculturation* to describe the effects of acculturation at the individual level of study. More recently, John Berry and his colleagues (e.g., Segall, Dasen, Berry, & Poortinga, 1999) developed a model of acculturation in which one continuum represents *"contact and participation* (to what extent should [people] become involved in other cultural groups, or remain primarily among themselves)" and another continuum representing *"cultural maintenance* (to what extent are cultural identity and characteristics considered to be important, and their maintenance striven for)" (p. 305).

Associated with the concept of acculturation is the concept of *enculturation*. Herskovits (1948) described enculturation as the process of socialization to and maintenance of the norms of one's indigenous culture, including the salient values, ideas, and concepts. Based on this description, it can be explained that the "cultural maintenance" process that is mentioned by Berry and his colleagues as a part of acculturation may be better represented with this broader terminology of enculturation. Although Segall et al.'s (1999) characterization of acculturation in terms of cultural maintenance may work well for immigrant Asian Americans who have been socialized into their Asian cultural norms before arriving in the United States, it may not accurately describe the experiences of Asian Americans who were born in the United States. These Asian Americans, particularly individuals who are several generations removed from immigration, may have never been fully enculturated into the Asian ethnic group's cultural norms by their parents and family who may also be U.S.-born. For these persons, the application of the "cultural maintenance" process may not be appropriate. In addition, these persons may become socialized to their Asian heritage more fully later in life and hence engage in the process of enculturation during that time. For these reasons, the term *enculturation* offers a more comprehensive description of incorporating and maintaining one's ethnic cultural norms, in comparison to the "cultural maintenance" concept within the acculturation construct. Furthermore, an added benefit of using the term enculturation is that it places an equal level of focus on the process of socializing into and retaining one's Asian cultural norms as compared to the process of adapting to and maintaining the norms of the U.S. culture.

Consistent with this explanation, it has been proposed that enculturation be used to describe the process of (re)socializing into and maintaining the norms of the indigenous culture and acculturation be used to describe the process of adapting to the norms of the dominant culture (Kim & Abreu, 2001). For Asian Americans, therefore, acculturation refers to the process of adapting to the norms of the U.S. culture, and enculturation refers to the process of becoming socialized into and maintaining the norms of the Asian culture. Current theories of acculturation and enculturation suggest that Asian Americans who are farther removed from immigration will adhere to the mainstream U.S. cultural norms more strongly than Asian Americans who are recent immigrants (Kim, Atkinson, & Umemoto, 2001). On the other hand, Asian Americans who are closer to immigration will adhere to Asian cultural norms more strongly than their counterparts who are several generations removed from immigration.

Early acculturation theorists (Berry & Annis, 1974; Szapocznik, Scopetta, Kurtines, & Aranalde, 1978) conceptualized acculturation and enculturation as processes that take place along a single, or unilinear, continuum. According to this model, adaptation occurs when a person moves from one end of a continuum, reflecting involvement in the culture of origin (i.e., enculturation), to the other end of the same continuum, reflecting involvement in the host culture (i.e., acculturation). Szapocznik, Kurtines, and Fernandez (1980) noted that these theories

> conceptualized immigrants as adopting host-culture behavior and values while simultaneously discarding those attributes of their culture of origin. Thus, acculturation has been viewed as a process in which there is an inverse linear relationship between an individual's involvement with his/her original and host cultures. (p. 353)

A number of scholars (Mendoza, 1984, 1989; Padilla, 1980; Ramirez, 1984; Szapocznik & Kurtines, 1980) have pointed out the limitations of this unilinear model, specifically noting its inability to represent true biculturalism. Biculturalism refers to having strong adherence to both the Asian and dominant U.S. cultural norms. Szapocznik and Kurtines (1980) noted that biculturalism would be an important aspect of acculturation because the pre-existence of a minority community would lead to the process of an individual retaining the culture of origin while accommodating to the host culture. Given that there are already large communities of Asian Americans across the country and new immigrants who continue to join these communities, the concept of biculturalism is particular relevant.

Recognizing this important limitation of the unilinear model, John Berry and his colleagues (Berry, 1990, 1994; Berry & Kim, 1988; Berry, Kim, Power, Young, & Bajaki, 1989; Berry, Trimble, & Olmeda, 1986) developed

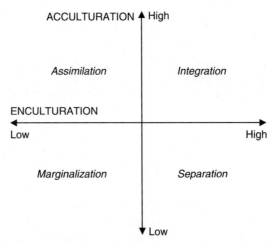

FIGURE **1** Bilinear Model of Adaptation
Adapted from Berry (1990, 1994).

a bilinear model in which one linearity represents acculturation and another linearity represents enculturation. Research examining the validity of this bilinear model has found the model to be far superior to the unilinear model (Ryder, Alden, & Paulhus, 2000; Miller, 2007). Based on the bilinear model, Berry and his colleagues theorized the following four acculturation "attitudes" based on combining either high or low levels of each linearity: *Integration*, *Assimilation*, *Separation*, and *Marginalization*; see Figure 1.

Integration occurs when individuals become proficient in the culture of the dominant group while retaining proficiency in the indigenous culture. People in this status are both highly acculturated and strongly enculturated. Asian Americans in this status may be most healthy because it allows them to hold cultural norms that are functional in both European and Asian American cultures while being able to reconcile any conflicts that arise between the two cultural systems. Consider Jennifer, a second-generation Laotian American college student in her final year as a business administration major. Jennifer's parents immigrated in their early twenties and married just after college. They raised Jennifer to be fluent in the majority culture while respecting and adhering to the cultural norms of the Laotian culture. Jennifer was an active member of the Girls Scouts while also a student at a Laotian language school in the community. Although Jennifer initially rejected the customs of the Laotian culture, particularly during her middle school years (e.g., she did not like attending the language school), she has now become fully accepting of and fluent in this culture. Currently, she is the president of Laotian Student Union on her campus and actively partici-pates in Laotian cultural festivals. She also volunteers as a translator for a community agency that serves newly-arrived Laotian immigrants. In terms of her interaction with dominant society, Jennifer also is fluent in the majority culture (e.g., she is an officer for one of the oldest and largest sororities in the country). She plans to eventually earn a MBA and then become a CEO of a U.S. company doing international business with Laos and other Southeast Asian countries.

- For people like Jennifer, how successful do you think they will be in life?
- What are the major areas of strengths for people like Jennifer?
- What attitudes and skills do people like Jennifer have that will enable them to be successful in life?

Assimilation, on the other hand, occurs when an individual absorbs the culture of the dominant group while rejecting the indigenous culture. Individuals in this status are highly acculturated but not enculturated. Asian Americans in this status typically maintain cultural norms that are impor-tant in the dominant U.S. culture but have no interest in adhering to Asian cultural norms. Consider Phil, a third-generation Japanese American gay man in his thirties who works as a graphic designer for a large advertising firm. Phil came out to his family and friends in his early twenties. Unfortu-nately, although his friends accepted Phil's sexual identity, his family, who adheres to traditional Japanese cultural norms, rejected him. His family simply could not believe that Phil could be attracted to other men. Conse-quently, Phil moved out of his family's home and began to live on his own while finishing up his college degree. Currently, Phil socializes mainly with non-Asian Americans, typically with European Americans who are accept-ing of Phil's identity. Incidentally, there is research showing that Asian Americans tend not to have positive perceptions of same-sex relation-ships. For example, in a study of 397 college students in Hawai'i, Japanese, Filipino, and Chinese Americans were found to be significantly more distancing toward persons in same-sex relations in comparison to European Americans (Kim, D'Andrea, Sahu, & Gaughen, 1998). In addition, Chinese and Japanese Americans were found to have significantly less accurate information about homosexuality than did European Americans (Kim et al., 1998).

Separation occurs when an individual is not interested in learning the culture of the dominant group and wants only to maintain and perpetuate the culture of origin. Individuals in this status are strongly enculturated but not acculturated. Asian Americans in this status typically maintain Asian cultural norms but have no interest in adhering to the dominant U.S. cultural norms. Consider Hassan, a first-generation Pakistani American engineer in his late forties who immigrated five years ago with his wife and lives in a Pakistani enclave in a large city. Upon arrival to the United States, Hassan was unable to find an engineering position with a mainstream firm due to

(continues)

(continued)

his limited English proficiency. As a result, Hassan, with the help of his wife, opened a small grocery store specializing in goods from Pakistan and serving mainly other Pakistani Americans. Although Hassan is disappointed about being unable to work as an engineer, he is happy that the store is doing well. Hassan is an active member of the local mosque, and he has strong ties with the local Pakistani American community whom he sought out soon after arriving in the area. He is currently in the process of bringing his elderly parents over from Islamabad to stay with him and his wife. Given his work and the area of residence, Hassan seldom has contact with members of the dominant group.

Finally, marginalization represents the attitude of an individual with no interest in maintaining or acquiring proficiency in any culture, dominant or indigenous. Individuals in this status are neither acculturated nor enculturated. Marginalization is perhaps the most problematic of the four statuses because marginalized Asian Americans will adhere to neither cultural systems and tend to reject both sets of norms. Consider Moua, a Hmong American in his early teens who lives in a Midwestern state. Moua was born in a refugee camp in Thailand before arriving in the United States just two years ago. Since his arrival Moua has had difficulty adjusting to the new life here. Although he had some English lessons in the camp, he is not proficient in it and has had a lot of trouble communicating with others at school. Moua feels no connection to school or any aspects of the U.S. culture. Consequently, Moua has tried to avoid interacting with members of the majority group. Unfortunately, Moua also does not feel any connection to the Hmong culture. Given that he was raised in a refugee camp, where his parents were busy trying to survive and where the Hmong culture was not maintained, Moua did not have good socialization experiences with this culture. As a result, Moua does not feel close to either the Hmong or the U.S. culture. Adding to these problems is that Moua's family also lives in poverty. Given the traumas suffered during the Vietnam War, Moua's father suffers from post-traumatic stress disorder and is unable to work. Moua's mother is the only income earner and works at a job that pays minimum wage. Recently, Moua's parents have been very worried because Moua is beginning to come home late and hang out with the "wrong crowd."

As discussed above, the Integration (or Biculturalism) status may be the healthiest status for Asian Americans. In addition, the literature on biculturalism suggests that individuals who can effectively function in both the indigenous and dominant cultures may exhibit increased cognitive functioning and mental health (LaFromboise, Coleman, and Gerton, 1993). LaFromboise et al. (1993) used the term *bicultural competence* to describe this process in which individuals are able to successfully meet the demands of two distinct cultures. They described bicultural competence as including (a) knowledge of cultural beliefs and values of both cultures, (b) positive attitudes toward both groups,

(c) bicultural efficacy, or belief that one can live in a satisfying manner within both cultures without sacrificing one's cultural identity, (d) communication ability in both cultures, (e) role repertoire, or the range of culturally appropriate behaviors, and (f) a sense of being grounded in both cultures. LaFromboise et al. noted that individuals may experience difficulties adjusting to the different and sometimes opposing demands, but when they are able to obtain these skills they may be able to increase their performance in vocational and academic endeavors. Consistent with these ideas, research has shown that high levels of both acculturation and enculturation are positively associated with Asian Americans feeling good about their ethnic group (Omizo, Kim, & Abel, 2008) and being members of the group (Kim & Omizo, 2005; Kim & Omizo, 2006).

In examining levels of acculturation and enculturation, it is important to consider various ways in which the two types of adherence can be assessed. Szapocznik et al. (1978) first elaborated on ways of assessing acculturation and enculturation by proposing that it involved changes in two personal dimensions: behaviors and values. The behavioral dimension of acculturation includes language use and participation in various cultural activities (e.g., food consumption), while the values dimension reflects relational style, person-nature relationships, beliefs about human nature, and time orientation. Padilla (1980) further expanded the conceptualization of acculturation by suggesting that this process also involved cultural awareness and ethnic loyalty. Cultural awareness refers to an individual's attunement to the cultural manifestations of native and host cultures. Ethnic loyalty, on the other hand, is an indication of preferences for one culture over the other, and includes an individual's level of ethnic pride and identity.

Definitions of acculturation have continued to grow progressively more integrative and comprehensive (e.g., Berry, 1980; Cuellar, Arnold, & Maldonado, 1995). For example, Berry (1980) identified six dimensions of psychological functioning directly affected by acculturation: language, cognitive styles, personality, identity, attitudes, and acculturative stress. Berry posited that as an individual moves through the acculturation process, changes occurred in each of these areas. Later, Cuellar et al. (1995) defined acculturation in terms of changes at three levels of functioning: behavioral, affective, and cognitive. They state

> The behavioral level includes many types of behaviors, including verbal behavior or language. Language development obviously includes aspects beyond the behavioral and is understood to include cognitive aspects and related processes. Also at the behavioral level are customs, foods, and such cultural expressions as the music one chooses to listen to or dance to. At the affective level are the emotions that have cultural connections. For example, the way a person feels about important aspects of identity, the symbols one loves or hates, and the meaning one attaches to itself are all culturally based. At the cognitive level are beliefs about male/female roles, ideas about illness, attitudes toward illness, and fundamental values. (p. 281)

In a review of scales designed to assess acculturation and enculturation, Kim and Abreu (2001) analyzed the item contents of 33 instruments and found them to be consistent with the conceptual framework of Cuellar et al. (1995). Specifically, Kim and Abreu found that the items could be categorized into one of the following four dimensions: behavior, values, knowledge, and cultural identity. Behavior is a dimension along the Cuellar et al.'s behavioral level of functioning and refers to friendship choice, preferences for television programs and reading, participation in cultural activities, contact with indigenous culture (e.g., time spent in the country of origin), language use, food choice, and music preference. Along the cognitive level of functioning, Kim and Abreu identified two dimensions, values and knowledge. The value dimension refers to attitudes and beliefs about social relations, cultural customs, and cultural traditions, along with gender roles and attitudes and ideas about health and illness. The knowledge dimension refers to culturally specific information such as names of historical leaders in the culture of origin and the dominant culture, and historical significance of culturally specific activities. Along the affective level of functioning, Kim and Abreu proposed the inclusion of cultural identity. Cultural identify refers to attitudes toward one's cultural identification (e.g., preferred name is in Spanish), attitudes toward indigenous and dominant groups (e.g., feelings of shame towards the indigenous culture and pride towards the dominant group), and level of comfort towards people of indigenous and dominant groups.

Using these dimensions, counselors can assess levels of acculturation and enculturation of their Asian American clients. For instance, along the behavioral dimension, a first-generation Korean American adult who prefers to watch Korean-language television channels and eat Korean food over watching U.S. channels and eating American food could be said to be strongly enculturated but not very acculturated. A third-generation Laotian American teenager who prefers to listen to U.S. music over Laotian music could be said to be strongly acculturated but minimally enculturated. On the other hand, a second-generation Asian Indian young adult who equally prefers American and Indian food and music could be said to be bicultural (or integrationist). Along the dimension of values, a first-generation Taiwanese American grandfather who strongly adheres to Asian cultural values but eschews U.S. values could be said to be strongly enculturated but not acculturated. But a fifth-generation Japanese American adult who strongly adheres to U.S. cultural values but does not endorse any Asian values could be said to be highly acculturated but not enculturated. Along the knowledge dimension, a first-generation Chinese American grandmother who understands the significance of fireworks and dragon dance during the Chinese New Year can be said to be highly enculturated. A fifth-generation Filipino American elderly person who understands the history behind the U.S. holiday of Thanksgiving can be said to be highly acculturated. On the other hand, a second-generation Vietnamese American adult who understands the importance of both the Tet celebration and the Fourth of July can be said to be both highly enculturated and acculturated, or bicultural. Lastly, along the cultural identity dimension, a Pakistani American adult who prefers to be called by his indigenous name could be said to be strongly enculturated, whereas an Asian Indian American adult who prefers to be called only by his American name can be said to be highly acculturated.

RACIAL AND ETHNIC IDENTITY DEVELOPMENT

The theory of racial and ethnic identity development is another useful tool to examine the variability that exists among Asian Americans. Among the various models of this theory, Atkinson's (2004) Minority Identity Development (MID) model might be most useful in illustrating the varied experiences of Asian Americans. As explained by these authors, the MID model "defines five stages of development that oppressed people may experience as they struggle to understand themselves in terms of their own minority culture and the oppressive relationship between the [minority and majority] cultures" (p. 34). The five stages are as follows: *Conformity*, *Dissonance*, *Resistance and Immersion*, *Introspection*, and *Synergistic Articulation and Awareness*. Atkinson pointed out that the five stages represent a continuous process in which one stage tends to blend with the next stage.

According to the MID model, Asian Americans who are in the Conformity stage will have preference over the dominant U.S. cultural values over Asian values. Consider Rosalie, a second-generation Filipino American in her early 20s. Having grown up in a predominantly European American community, Rosalie views European Americans as role models whose value system and resulting lifestyles should be followed. On the other hand, Rosalie views Asian cultural values to be undesirable and inferior, and rejects them. Although she is not sure why she feels this way, she has always had negative views about Asian Americans. Like Rosalie, Asian Americans in the Conformity stage will have self- and group-depreciating attitudes, while viewing the European American group with positive attitudes. In addition, because they reject their status as members of a minority group, these Asian Americans will have discriminatory attitudes toward other minority groups.

Asian Americans who are in the Dissonance stage may have reached this stage gradually or as a result of a monumental event. An example of a critical event for a Japanese American, for instance, might be learning in a history course that thousands of Japanese Americans were unjustly placed in internment camps during World War II, but that many of these Japanese Americans joined the 442nd Regimental Combat Team that fought so courageously for the United States in Europe. In the case of Rosalie, the Filipina American described above, a critical event for her might be learning that thousands of Filipinos in the past served bravely in the U.S. Navy but were not eligible for U.S. citizenship. Asian Americans in this stage are faced with information that brings positive light to their Asian American group as well as negative light to the European American group. As a result, these individuals are now forced to evaluate their attitudes toward the Asian and European American groups and to reconcile these dissonant pieces of information. Hence, Asian Americans in this stage are in a state of

(continues)

(continued)

conflict between self- and group-depreciating attitudes and self- and group-appreciating attitudes with respect to the Asian American group. Similarly, they are in a state of conflict over their positive and negative attitudes toward the European American and other minority groups.

According to the MID model, Asian Americans in the Dissonance stage may eventually move to the Resistance and Immersion stage, which is characterized by a complete endorsement of the Asian cultural values and a complete rejection of the European American values. In the case of Rosalie, if she enters this stage, she will actively seek and explore her Filipino American history and culture that enhances her sense of identity and worth. She will look for information about Filipino Americans in the United States and attend cultural events that document how they have contributed to this country. Characteristics defining Filipino Americans change from being sources of shame and disgust to being symbols of pride and honor. As a result, Rosalie and other Asian Americans like her have an appreciating attitude about their Asian American groups, while they hold negative attitudes toward the European American group. In terms of their attitudes toward other minority groups, Asian Americans in this stage experience feelings of empathy and a growing sense of camaraderie with members of other minority groups.

In the Introspection stage, Asian Americans experience feelings of discontent and discomfort with the views held in the Resistance and Immersion stage. For example, Rosalie may begin to feel more comfortable with her own sense of identity as a Filipino American and question the basis for her views in the previous stage. There is a growing awareness that perhaps not everything about the Filipino American group is good and everything about the European American group is bad. Rosalie and other Asian Americans in the introspection stage may begin to have concerns about their overwhelming positive view of the Asian American groups and the ethnocentric basis for judging others. They also may begin to recognize the utility of many European American cultural elements but be uncertain about whether to incorporate such elements into their own cultural norms.

Finally, Asian Americans in the Synergistic stage experience a sense of self-fulfillment with regards to their own identity. According to Atkinson (2004), the conflict and discomfort that was experienced during the Introspection stage have been reconciled, allowing for greater individual control and flexibility. For Rosalie and others like her, cultural values of both Asian and European American cultures are examined and evaluated objectively, and the desire to eliminate oppression becomes an important motivation for their own behavior. Rosalie may become more critical in how she evaluates the race dynamics in the United States and consider it in a much more complex and thoughtful manner.

The MID model can be particularly useful in helping counselors to understand the unique experiences of Asian American clients. As such, Atkinson (2004) described three ways in which the model can be helpful. First, the model can sensitize counselors to the role oppression plays in Asian Americans' identity development. Second, the model can also help counselors to appreciate the differences that can exist between Asian Americans with respect to their identity. Third, the model describes the potential Asian Americans have for changing their sense of identity.

ADHERENCE TO ASIAN CULTURAL VALUES

An important similarity between the theory of acculturation and enculturation and the MID model is their focus on cultural values as a way to discern the experiences of Asian Americans and their cultural socialization. Indeed, Kluckhohn (1951) made values a central component of his definition of culture. He noted,

> Culture consists in patterned ways of thinking, feeling and reacting, acquired and transmitted by symbols, constituting the distinctive achievements of human groups, including their embodiments in artifacts; the essential core of culture consists of traditional (i.e., historically derived and selected) ideas and especially their values. (p. 86)

Also, knowing clients' adherence to various cultural values can provide important information in regards to how they function psychologically and will respond to counseling. It can be argued that having a good understanding of clients' cultural values may be more important than having a good understanding of their behavioral norms, knowledge level, and cultural identity status. For example, imagine working with a first-generation Thai client who immigrated to the United States five years ago. The client seems to you to be highly acculturated in terms of his behavior (e.g., speaks English well), knowledge about the United States (e.g., can discuss the political history of the United States), and his cultural identity (e.g., prefers to be called by his English name). However, you soon find out that he is strongly enculturated in terms of values (e.g., strongly adheres to the Asian norms of collectivism, conformity to norms, and filial piety). You then recognize that if you do not attend to his cultural values, you might have incorrectly concluded that he was highly acculturated. Also you realize that with these types of clients, their psychological functioning would be more closely dictated by their values rather than their display of other dimensions of general functioning. In other words, because psychological functioning, such as one's attitudes and worldview, are closely related to one's value system, having a good understanding of clients' cultural values is important. Without the consideration of cultural values, you may have had the misperception that the client is highly acculturated, although in fact there are important characteristics that suggest a high level of values enculturation.

What follows is a review of the literature on Asian cultural values, with a focus on how these values may influence the worldviews of Asian Americans. I decided to focus on Asian values because they can serve as an important basis for determining one's level of enculturation. Also, examining Asian American client's adherence to Asian values can serve as a good starting point for determining the person's level of acculturation. For example, if a counselor learns that a client does not endorse a particular Asian cultural value, the counselor can then explore whether the client might endorse a contrasting value in the dominant U.S. culture. This might allow the counselor to explore the client's level of values acculturation and help the client discover his or her identity. Before continuing, I need to reemphasize that it is very important to keep in mind the within-group variability with these values and that not all Asian Americans will adhere equally to these values. For Asian Americans who are highly enculturated, the values described below will be salient, but for Asian Americans who are low enculturated, these values may not be relevant to their lives. Also, there are important differences between Asian American ethnic groups on their levels of adherence to these values. More information about this follows this section.

Many writers have described the various aspects of traditional Asian cultural values and their effects on Asian Americans across diverse ethnic groups (e.g., Chen, 1982; Fernandez, 1988; Ho, 1987; Kaneshige, 1973; Kitano & Matsushima, 1981; Morrow, 1989; Sue & Sue, 2003; Tinloy, 1978; Tomita, 1994; Uba, 1994). Kim et al. (2001) after a review of this literature presented the following summary. Asian Americans' self-worth and self-identity are strongly tied to their family's achievements, as dictated by traditional Asian cultural values. When members of Asian American families achieve success, it usually reflects positively on the entire family. Conversely, when Asian Americans fail at a task or engage in inappropriate social behavior, the entire family often shares in the same embarrassment and loss of face. Thus, one of the major responsibilities of all family members is to avoid bringing shame and loss of face to the family. The fear of losing face can be a powerful motivating force for an Asian American to conform to the family's expectations and often may be used to suppress deviation from family norms.

The roles of family members in Asian American families can be highly interdependent, rigidly defined, and strictly adhered to, as dictated by traditional Asian cultural values. The family structure may be arranged so that these roles do not interfere with each other, thus minimizing any possible role conflicts between family members. The father traditionally is the head of the household among many Asian American families. The mother traditionally is recognized as the nurturant caretaker of both her husband and children. The son's primary allegiance is to the family into which he is born; being a good husband or father is secondary to his duty as a son. On the other hand, the traditional role of the daughters is to perform domestic duties and to be subservient to the males in the family.

Allegiance to the parents, or filial piety, is strongly valued in traditional Asian cultures. Filial piety is characterized by respect, honor, fidelity, devotion, dutifulness, and sacrifice on the part of children for their parents. Filial piety demands unquestioning obedience to parents as well as concern for and understanding of their needs and wishes with the intention of comforting them. In addition to respect for parents, ancestors and elders are viewed with great reverence and respect. Also, Asian Americans who adhere strongly to Asian cultural values tend to defer to authority figures, including parents and elders, for decision making and problem resolution.

The Confucian value of interpersonal harmony can play a significant role in Asian Americans' communication style and interpersonal behavior. Following Confucius' teachings, Asian Americans may aspire to be patient, gentle, well-mannered, and cooperative. They also may attempt to blend in with the group rather than distinguish themselves through behaviors that stand out from the group. The Asian values of personal restraint and reservation underlie much of Asian American expressive behavior. When interacting with others, Asian Americans may tend to be accommodating, conciliatory, and receptive, rather than confrontational. They typically refrain from being verbal, preferring a passive communication style, and tend to refrain from openly challenging others' perspectives in order to maintain interpersonal harmony. On the other hand, Asian Americans often use nonverbal communication processes, including gestures and facial expressions, to convey feelings nonverbally during both conversation and silence.

The traditional Asian culture encourages the suppression of emotional conflicts and discourages the full expression of emotions. Thus, many Asian Americans are taught to have self-control and to exercise restraint when experiencing potentially disruptive emotions. These cultural values force many Asian Americans to be reticent in their interpersonal communication style. Also for traditional Asian Americans, self-effacement, modesty, discretion, and humility are highly valued. Asian Americans are discouraged from appearing bumptious by talking about their accomplishments or expressing their opinions and encouraged to be humble and modest. They may not want to seem boastful or self-centered because this also could negatively reflect the family.

Despite the relatively large number of articles that have been published describing these Asian cultural values and their possible effects on the behaviors of Asian Americans, little research had been done to empirically examine the presence of these cultural values among Asian Americans (Uba, 1994). An exception is a study by Kim et al. (1999), who in developing the *Asian Values Scale* attempted to empirically identify Asian cultural values and delineate more closely the various dimensions of Asian cultural values, as perceived by Asian Americans in the United States.

Kim et al. (1999) identified the dimensions of Asian cultural values by using a three-stage research process: a) a review of the literature on Asian cultural values; b) a nation-wide survey of Asian American psychologists; and c) three focus-group discussions with Asian American participants. The literature review covered journal articles, books, book chapters, and dissertations on Asian cultural values; this review accessed the body of literature that is summarized above. For the survey of psychologists, 103 Asian American members of APA's Division 45 were identified by their surnames from the Membership Directory and sent a questionnaire packet. Twenty-eight Asian American psychologists and their associates returned the response form resulting in additional value statements that were collated and categorized under the Asian value dimensions generated from the literature review. Two one-hour focus discussion groups, comprising doctoral Asian American students in psychology, were used to generate additional Asian cultural value dimensions and statements describing each dimension; the participants in the groups included one Asian

Indian American, three Chinese Americans, and five Korean Americans. The third focus discussion group, comprising three psychology doctoral Asian American students, determined the accuracy of the pairings between the value dimensions and their corresponding statements and identified additional dimensions that had not been identified during the previous step; the participants in the group were one Burmese American, one Chinese American, and one Korean American. These procedures generated a total of 14 value dimensions with 202 items (see Kim, Atkinson, et al., 1999 for more details).

The following brief description of Asian values is organized according to the 14 value domains derived by Kim et al. (1999). The specific value statements identified by Kim et al. are used to describe each domain.

Ability to Resolve Psychological Problems

Each individual should be able to resolve psychological problems on his/her own. One should use one's inner resources and willpower to resolve psychological problems. Psychological problems are best dealt with, and mental health best maintained, by moderating one's emotions and behavior, controlling morbid thoughts, and seeking inner peace. One should overcome distress by oneself; asking others for psychological help is a sign of weakness.

Avoidance of Family Shame

Family reputation is a primary social concern. The worst thing an individual can do is to disgrace her/his family reputation. The failure of any individual family member reflects negatively on the family as a whole. Breaking family traditions and norms, defaulting on duties and obligations to the family, manifesting mental health problems, and failing to achieve academically and occupationally are ways that individuals can disgrace their family.

Collectivism

Individuals should feel a strong sense of attachment to the group to which they belong, and should think about the welfare of the group before their own welfare. Group interests and goals should be promoted over individual interests and goals. Similarly, an individual's obligations and duties to the group are more important than individual rights. One should be interdependent with other members of the group; working on a task with others is better than working on it by oneself. Spending time with one's group is preferable to spending time alone.

Conformity to Family and Social Norms and Expectations

Conforming to familial and societal norms is important; one should not deviate from these norms. It is important to follow and conform to the expectations that one's family and the society have for one. Individuals should not make waves and should avoid disrupting the status quo.

Deference to Authority Figures

Authority figures are deserving of respect. Individuals with higher education should receive greater respect than those with less education. One should be less verbal and listen more in the presence of authority figures because one can learn from them. Individuals should not question a person in a position of authority and never refer to an authority figure by their first name. Authority figures are in a position to evaluate an individual, never the other way around.

Educational and Occupational Achievement

Educational and occupational achievement should be an individual's top priorities. Success in life is defined in terms of one's academic and career accomplishments. Working hard is the way an individual can become academically and occupationally successful. Therefore hard work and perseverance in school and on the job are virtues. Complete devotion to one's studies will pay off later and will make one's parents proud.

Filial Piety

Children are expected to manifest unquestioning obedience to their parents. Children should never talk back to their parents, go against their parents' wishes, or question the authority of their parents. Parental love is usually not openly expressed but should be implicitly understood. Adult children are expected to take care of their aging parents, especially when the parents are unable to take care of themselves. Children should not place their parents in retirement or nursing homes.

Importance of Family

Individual family members feel a strong sense of obligation to the family as a whole and a commitment to maintaining family well-being. Interdependence and mutual trust are important family values. Honor and duty to one's family are very important, more important than one's own fame and power; personal accomplishment is interpreted as family achievement. In fact, individual family members are expected to make sacrifices for the family. Individual members are also expected to follow the role expectations set by their family as a whole.

Maintenance of Interpersonal Harmony

In a disagreement, one should overlook differences in an effort to maintain harmony. One should always try to be accommodating and conciliatory and never directly confrontational. Non-verbal communication plays an important part in maintaining interpersonal harmony. An individual should never express his or her feelings at the expense of maintaining harmony. One should not say things that may offend another person or that would cause the other person to lose face. In fact, one should always provide a dignified way for the other person to save face.

Placing Other's Needs ahead of One's Own

An individual should consider the needs of others before considering one's own. One should anticipate and be aware of the needs of others and not inconvenience them. Over-asserting one's own needs is a sign of immaturity. An individual should look out for other people's feelings and observe his or her behavior to prevent others from feeling uncomfortable.

Reciprocity

An individual should repay another person's favor, that is, repay those people who have helped or provided assistance to the individual. Thus, when one receives a gift, that person should reciprocate with a gift of equal or greater value. Reciprocity works both ways, and when one does favors for others, he or she should accept favors in return. In this vein, friends should take turns paying for each other. There is a direct relationship between how well one treats others and how well one is treated.

Respect for Elders and Ancestors

Ancestors and elders should be viewed with reverence and respect; children should honor their elders and ancestors. Elders have more wisdom and deserve more respect than young people. Young people should avoid bringing displeasure to their elders. Young people should never confront their elders, talk back to them, or go directly against their wishes.

Self-Control and Restraint

One should exercise restraint when experiencing strong emotions. It is better to hold your pain, suffering, and anger inside than to express them. Neither strong positive emotions nor strong negative emotions should be expressed. Instead, one should remain reserved and tranquil. The ability to control emotions is a sign of strength.

Self-Effacement

It is important to minimize or depreciate one's own achievements. One should be humble, modest, and not boastful. It is inappropriate to draw attention to oneself. In fact, individuals should be discouraged from talking about their accomplishments. Individuals should avoid thinking that they are better than others. Instead, accomplishments should be attributed to the support they have received from others.

The 14 value dimensions identified by Kim et al. (1999) represent a support for and an expansion of the literature on Asian cultural values. In reviewing these values, it is important to note that these dimensions are related to each other. A common thread among the dimensions is Confucianism and Buddhism, a set of philosophical and religious beliefs that promote the values of interpersonal harmony, knowledge and acceptance of one's place in society and the family, obedience, and orientation toward the group (Uba, 1994). In addition to this conceptual interrelationship between the value dimensions, Kim, Yang, Atkinson, Wolfe, and Hong (2001) demonstrated empirically, through the use of confirmatory factor analysis and factorial invariance analysis of structural equation modeling, that many of these value dimensions serve as good statistical indicators of an overarching Asian cultural values construct. This finding provides further evidence for the interrelatedness among the dimensions of Asian cultural values and suggests that a person's adherence to some of the Asian cultural value dimensions can be indicative of that person's adherence to other Asian cultural value dimensions, albeit to different degrees (Kim et al. 1999).

CULTURAL VALUES, SIMILARITIES, AND DIFFERENCES ACROSS ASIAN ETHNIC GROUPS

Although these cultural values are commonly observed among Asian Americans, it is important to keep in mind that not all Asian Americans will endorse them equally. As pointed out earlier, these values are more salient and adhered to by those who are psychologically closer to the Asian culture (e.g., a recent immigrant from Thailand) than those who are farther removed from the Asian culture (e.g., a sixth-generation Japanese American). Hence, these values should serve as a way to determine the level of enculturation among Asian Americans, rather than a tool to stereotype them into a uniform set of characteristics.

Consistent with this thinking, a recent study by Kim et al. (2001) found significant similarities and differences among Chinese, Filipino, Japanese, and Korean Americans on their adherence to some of these values. In their study, Kim et al. (2001) used the Asian Values Scale (AVS; Kim et al., 1999), which is a measure of adherence to the following Asian cultural values: collectivism, conformity to norms, emotional self-control, family recognition through achievement, filial piety, and humility. In terms of similarities, the results of the study indicated that the members of all four ethnic groups attributed similar meanings to the six value dimensions. This finding suggests that these values dimensions are commonly perceived and defined by various groups of Asian Americans. This finding is important in that it supports the notion that these cultural values are salient to Asian Americans in general and not unique to only certain cultures. However, this finding may not be surprising when considering that the philosophical and religious sources for these values, namely Confucianism and Buddhism, can be found across the Asian continent (Uba, 1994).

In terms of differences, Kim et al. (2001) found that Filipino Americans indicated (a) less adherence to emotional self-control than the other three groups, (b) less adherence to family recognition through achievement and filial piety than Japanese and Korean Americans, (c) less adherence to conformity to norms than Chinese and Japanese Americans, and (d) less adherence to collectivism than Japanese Americans. Also, Japanese Americans had higher adherence to conformity to norms than did Chinese Americans, and Japanese and Korean Americans had higher adherence to family recognition through achievement than did Chinese Americans. These findings are important because it suggests that although these value dimensions are commonly observed across the four groups, members of these groups endorse the values in a differential fashion.

However, these findings of differences are not surprising when considering the histories of the Philippines, China, Japan, and Korea in terms of various philosophical and religious influences. Although Buddhism and Confucian philosophy influenced all four groups, the unique religious and cultural influences exerted in the past by two colonial powers on the Filipinos have mitigated the Asian cultural value effects of Buddhism and Confucianism. Specifically, the Spanish conquistadors colonized the Philippines in 1521, which led to the rise of Catholicism as the new state religion and the ascension of Spaniards and Spanish mestizos (biracial Spanish and Filipino) to the ruling class. This led to changes in Filipino society as the Catholic Church discredited native Filipino priests and native Filipinos became second-class citizens. Also, the colonization of the Philippines by the United States in 1898 caused changes in Filipino society such as the adoption of the English language as the medium of communication in educational institutions that resulted in the transmission of American cultural values (Espiritu, 1995). Thus, it can be said that Filipino American culture is a mixture of Asian, Spanish, and American cultural influences in which values common in Confucian philosophy and Buddhism are tempered by values found in Spain and the United States. As for Chinese, Japanese, and Koreans, the influences of Buddhism and Confucian philosophy to a large extent have remained constant, with few modifications resulting from the infusion of Taoism in China, Christianity in South Korea, and Shintoism in Japan.

COMMUNICATION STYLES

Related to cultural values, effective counseling with Asian American clients involves a good understanding of communication norms and behaviors among these clients. A first consideration is language itself. Given the high number of foreign-born Asian Americans, there are many individuals with low English language proficiency. Obviously, this could become a barrier when counselors work with Asian American clients, and even in the presence of an interpreter, it could lead to inaccurate exchanges of information. Hence, counselors must take care when working with clients with low English proficiency to minimize misunderstandings.

A second consideration is how the information that is transmitted. Asian Americans tend to participate in "high-context" as opposed to "low-context" communication. In high-context communication, individuals expect the other person to infer information primarily from the context and knowledge of the communicator. Thus, high-context communication tends to be indirect and implicit. For example, two high-context communicators may accurately understand the communicated messages between each other without having all of the details spelled out. In contrast, individuals who employ low-context communication anticipate that information can be obtained from an explicit transmitted message. Thus, low-context communication tends to be direct and clear (Gudykunst, 2001). Consistent with these ideas, Park and Kim (2008) found that Asian Americans used a more high-context communication style of being indirect than European Americans. In addition, Asian Americans who adhered strongly to Asian cultural values tended to use less direct style such as being contentious and dramatic and used more indirect style such as inferring meaning.

Within the purview of the hierarchical social structure predominating traditional Asian cultures, high-context communication is pervasive. Asian Americans, particularly those who are highly enculturated, communicate according to "face," that is individual's projected images of themselves in social situations. High-context communication serves the purpose of maintaining and building face, where communication varies in regard to the relative social position of interacting members. For example, traditional Asian Americans would refer to a parent by their role, such as "father," rather than "you." Unlike European Americans, who tend to emphasize self-enhancement as a means of building face, Asian Americans, particularly those who are highly enculturated, are self-effacing and modest. For example, a European American might be encouraged in career counseling to describe her strengths. This may be culturally incongruent for traditional Asian Americans. In addition, while European Americans typically use humor to save face, traditional Asian Americans are usually apologetic. In sum, the following characterize traditional Asian American communication: being indirect, making inferences, using apology to maintain and build "face," acknowledging hierarchy in social situations, and being modest.

The importance of face in communication may translate into unique communication patterns when counselors work with Asian American clients, particularly those individuals who are highly enculturated. In terms of sequences of vocalizations and pauses, these individuals, compared to European Americans, may talk less at any one time (i.e., use fewer words) and have longer silences between vocalizations when communicating with other Asian Americans. However, when speaking with strangers, traditional Asian Americans might feel uncomfortable with silences because they may be anxious about the uncertainty of the norms and rules of communicating based on the stranger's cultural background. Traditional Asian Americans also tend to be polite in communication as they are considerate of others' feelings, foster mutual comfort, and build rapport. The degree to which traditional Asian Americans are polite also depends on the relative social position of the communicators; where individuals with higher social statuses are regarded with more politeness (Gudykunst, 2001). In addition, traditional Asian Americans are less likely to express emotion in communication due to the culturally high value placed on stoicism (Gudykunst, 2001).

SUMMARY AND CONCLUSIONS

This chapter's content focused on the constructs of acculturation and enculturation and racial and ethnic identity development that can serve as a useful conceptual basis for understanding the within-group variations among Asian Americans. Given the diversity of Asian Americans in terms of immigration history and generation status, gaining a good understanding of these constructs is critical for counselors to accurately conceptualize the experiences of Asian Americans in terms of their relations to the dominant and indigenous cultures. For example, it can be readily reasoned that the counseling needs of someone who is highly acculturated but low enculturated would be different than for someone who has low acculturation but high enculturation and highly enculturated. The next chapter will focus on the kinds of counseling services that may be helpful for these different types of Asian American clients.

Also, this chapter placed special attention on the cultural values that are commonly observed among Asian Americans, with an explanation of variations on the degree to which these values are adhered, and the related communication styles. Given that counseling is such a highly value-laden endeavor (see Sue & Sue, 2003) and emphasizes verbal communication, it is important for counselors to be especially aware of the values that clients bring with them to counseling, as well as the values that counselors bring to counseling, and how they influence the communication process in session. To the extent that there is a discrepancy between the values of the clients and those of counselors, the chance for a successful outcome may be diminished. Hence, it is important for counselors to be very aware of their own cultural values as a way to try to avoid having these values contaminate the counseling process. This issue also will be further explored in the next chapter.

CHAPTER 5

Counseling Dynamics and Interventions

In the previous chapters, I provided a demographic profile of Asian Americans and descriptions of their sociopolitical history, current status regarding oppression, resiliency and strength, and cultural systems related to mental health. The information in these chapters is intended to serve as the basis for understanding the psychological functioning of Asian Americans. In this chapter, I discuss how counselors can meet the psychological needs of Asian Americans based on this information. Specifically, the chapter contains information about (1) attitudes about seeking mental health services, (2) psychological assessment, (3) indigenous healing methods, (4) potential areas of conflict between Asian Americans' cultural values and conventional approaches to psychological treatment, (5) modification of conventional forms of counseling to meet the unique cultural needs, and (6) additional sources of mental health support.

In each of these sections, I include a clinical vignette that further illustrates the issues that are discussed. In addition, where available, I describe findings from research studies that bear on the issues. Throughout this chapter, special attention is placed on issues of acculturation and enculturation and racial and ethnic identity, because most multicultural counseling theory and research with Asian Americans have shown that these constructs are important in understanding the within-group variability among this group (Atkinson, 2004). In particular, adherence to Asian cultural values, a dimension of enculturation, is highlighted in the chapter. As you read this chapter, I invite you to consider the following questions.

- How can the information presented in the previous chapters help counselors to gain a more comprehensive psychological picture of Asian American clients?

- What are Asian Americans' attitudes about counseling and how are these attitudes influenced by Asian Americans' levels of acculturation and enculturation?

- What are the limitations of conventional counseling theories in meeting the needs of Asian Americans?

- What counseling strategies are useful when working with Asian Americans?

ATTITUDES ABOUT SEEKING MENTAL HEALTH SERVICES

Mental Health Service Utilization Patterns

Given the dramatic increase in the number of Asian Americans in the United States and based on anecdotal observations that they tend not to seek counseling services, mental health researchers have explored the rates of mental health service utilization among Asian Americans during the past few decades to see if these numbers are comparable to other cultural groups. In general, the results have supported the anecdotal observations that Asian Americans tend not seek psychological services. Snowden and Cheung (1990), based on a review of 1980 and 1981 nationwide survey data from the National Institute of Mental Health, found that Asian Americans had the lowest rates of admission into hospitals for mental health concerns among all racial and ethnic groups. Research studies using local samples also found underutilization of psychological services by Asian Americans living in California (Sue, Fujino, Hu, Takeuchi, & Zane, 1991; Sue & Kirk, 1975), Hawai'i (Kinzie & Tseng, 1978; Leong, 1994; Sue & Morishima, 1982), Washington (Sue, 1977; Sue & McKinney, 1975), and the West Coast in general (Sue & Sue, 1974). In particular, Sue and Morishima (1982) reviewed the records of psychiatric hospitalization in Hawai'i and found that Japanese, Chinese, and Filipino Americans were hospitalized at rates lower than European Americans. In a study of 14,000 clients over a three-year period at 17 community mental health centers in the greater Seattle area, Sue (1977) found that Asian Americans comprised only .7% of clients although they comprised 2.4% of the county's population. Similarly, a qualitative interview study found that Asian Americans would see a counselor only as the last resort, with friends and family as being first sources of support (Kim, Brenner, Liang, & Asay, 2003). In addition, a report by the U.S. Surgeon General concluded that Asian Americans tend to underutilize and prematurely terminate from mental health services, although their need for these services are no less than other racial groups (U.S. Department of Health and Human Services, 2001).

Interestingly, however, Snowden and Cheung (1990) also found that some Asian Americans in state and county mental hospitals required longer stays than all other ethnic groups, and those in Veterans Administration and private hospitals required longer stays than European Americans. When one considers this finding carefully in conjunction with that of Kim et al. (2003), it suggests that Asian Americans consider professional psychological help as the last resort and will seek help only when their problems have become extremely severe.

For other Asian American clients who seek help, however, there appears to be an increased tendency for premature termination from service. For example, Sue (1977) reported that 50% of Asian American clients failed to return for services after the initial intake interview, whereas the initial dropout rate for European Americans was 30%. According to the U.S. Surgeon General's report, this trend continues today (U.S. Department of Health and Human Services, 2001).

Perceptions of Mental Health Services and Their Providers

An initial review of these findings might suggest to counselors that Asian Americans experience mental health problems at a lower rate than other racial groups. Counselors also might believe that when Asian Americans do experience problems and seek psychological services, the problems tend to be minor in nature with only a few exceptions requiring extensive treatment at hospital settings. However, these speculations have been effectively dispelled by multicultural counseling scholars who argued that there are no particular reasons why Asian Americans, in comparison to other cultural groups, should have a lower rate of incidence for psychological problems (Atkinson, 2004; Sue, 1994). In fact, given the minority status of Asian Americans and their experiences of oppression in the United States (see Chapter 3), it seems reasonable to expect that the need for mental health services among this group will be greater than it will be for European Americans (Leong, Wagner, & Tata, 1995).

Therefore, other possible reasons must be considered to explain the finding that Asian Americans underutilize psychological services. One fruitful path of inquiry might be to consider that there may be some other factors within or outside the Asian American group that limit Asian Americans' use of psychological services. For example, one possibility is that there may be pre-existing and readily available therapeutic systems within Asian American communities. These systems may include a network of family members, respected elders, and practitioners of indigenous healing methods, all of which may be perceived as more credible sources of help than Western-based psychological services (Atkinson, 2004; Sue & Sue, 2003). In terms of the outside factors, it has been pointed out by many multicultural counseling scholars (e.g., Atkinson, 2004; Sue & Sue, 2003) that mainstream psychological service providers may lack cultural relevancy, sensitivity, and competency, which may discourage Asian Americans from seeking help from them.

While the presence of these factors is certainly possible (and will be further discussed later in this chapter), recent theoretical and research work has focused on two other within-group factors. These factors are (a) Asian Americans' lack of familiarity with conventional Western forms of psychological help, and (b) Asian cultural norms that discourage Asian Americans from seeking help from professional psychological service providers. As described in Chapter 4, a within-group variable that well reflects Asian Americans' familiarity with the dominant U.S. cultural norms in general, and specifically Western forms of psychological helping, is acculturation. Multicultural counseling scholars have suggested that Asian Americans who are not acculturated might perceive conventional psychological service to be overly foreign, not credible, or even threatening (Atkinson, 2004; Sue & Sue, 2003). In terms of the second factor, a within-group variable that reflects adherence to Asian cultural norms is enculturation (see Chapter 4). Multicultural counseling scholars have suggested that Asian Americans who are strongly enculturated may feel ashamed about having mental health problems and hesitate from revealing their problems with individuals outside their family such as a professional counselor (Atkinson, 2004; Sue, 1994).

Based on these ideas regarding acculturation and enculturation, multicultural counseling researchers have explored the influence of two attitudinal constructs that may be closely related to help-seeking behavior among Asian Americans. These constructs are *attitudes toward seeking professional psychological help* (Atkinson & Gim, 1989; Tata & Leong, 1994; Kim, 2007; Kim & Omizo, 2003) and *one's willingness to see a counselor for specific types of problems* (Atkinson, Lowe, & Matthews, 1995; Gim, Atkinson, & Whiteley, 1990; Kim & Omizo, 2003). The results of studies examining the relationship between acculturation and attitudes toward seeking professional psychological help have consistently indicated that less acculturated Asian Americans tend to have less favorable attitudes toward seeking professional psychological services than their more acculturated counterparts (Atkinson & Gim, 1989; Tata & Leong, 1994). This finding supports the idea that Asian Americans' underutilization of psychological services is related to their lack of familiarity with Western norms.

However, this picture becomes fuzzy when the construct of willingness to see a counselor is also considered. In contrast to the positive relationship for attitudes toward seeking professional psychological help, studies examining the relationship between Asian Americans' willingness to see a counselor and acculturation have shown that less acculturated Asian Americans tend to be *more* willing to see a counselor than their more acculturated counterparts. Given this inconsistency, the researchers tried to make sense of this finding by speculating that perhaps less acculturated Asian Americans, although they may hold negative attitudes toward seeking professional psychological help, may be willing to seek help from a counselor when they acknowledge the need for help (Gim et al., 1990; Atkinson, Whiteley, & Gim, 1990). The authors reasoned that perhaps some Asian cultural values such as *deference to authority figures* might cause traditional Asian Americans to ascribe a high level of credibility to highly educated professionals such as counselors. However, although this idea about the influence of Asian values is an interesting one, it is speculative at best because it must assume that not being acculturated is the same as being highly enculturated. If you recall, I discussed in Chapter 4 that there could be Asian Americans who are both low acculturated and low enculturated based on the bilinear model of acculturation and enculturation. Hence, the assumption that low acculturation is equal to high enculturation may not be valid.

Recognizing that low acculturation is not equivalent to high enculturation, recent efforts have been made to directly examine the relationship between enculturation and help-seeking attitudes. Although research on this issue is limited, a study by Kim and Omizo (2003) provides some initial insights into this issue. The authors investigated the relationships among Asian American college students' adherence to Asian cultural values, their attitudes toward seeking professional psychological services, and their willingness to see a counselor. Adherence to Asian values was measured using the Asian Values Scale (Kim, Atkinson, & Yang, 1999), which measures dimensions such as *collectivism, conformity to norms, emotional self-control, family recognition through achievement, filial piety,* and *humility.* After controlling for the effects of important demographic variables such as age, gender, generation since immigration, and previous counseling experience, the researchers found that high adherence to Asian cultural values was associated with both less positive attitudes toward seeking psychological help and less willingness to see a counselor. The results also showed that attitudes toward seeking professional psychological help mediated the relationship between adherence to Asian cultural values and willingness to see a counselor in general, and for personal problems and health problems, in particular. In other words, high adherence to Asian cultural values was related to less positive attitudes toward seeking professional psychological services, which, in turn, was related to decreased willingness to see a counselor for both general and specific concerns. In a follow-up study, Kim (2007) examined the relations between both values-enculturation and values-acculturation and attitudes toward seeking professional psychological help. Interestingly, when both acculturation and enculturation were examined simultaneously, a significant relation with help-seeking attitudes was found only for enculturation and not for acculturation. Hence, when adherence to Asian cultural values is directly assessed, the results support the idea that underutilization of psychological services among Asian Americans is related to Asian cultural norms, such as the value system, which discourage them from seeking conventional psychological services.

To summarize, all of these findings indicate that many Asian Americans underutilize psychological services because (a) they are not familiar with Western forms of helping, and (b) they adhere strongly to Asian cultural norms, specifically cultural values, that discourage Asian Americans from seeking outside help. Based on these findings, a number of counseling implications can be identified. First, given the lack of positive attitudes toward seeking professional psychological help by many Asian Americans, particularly those who are strongly enculturated or not acculturated, counselors might need to conduct more outreach services. Perhaps educational materials describing the potential benefits of psychological services can be developed for and distributed to Asian Americans in various community contexts (e.g., work, school). Also, counselors might develop informational materials to help Asian Americans cope with the stigma surrounding psychological problems and normalize the act of seeking help from a counselor. In these activities, it would be helpful for counselors to consult with other Asian American helping professionals who can suggest ways to maximize the effectiveness of these outreach efforts.

Second, mental health agencies should consider hiring Asian American counselors so that they can serve to attract Asian American clientele. This suggestion is especially appropriate if the agencies are located in communities with a large proportion of Asian Americans. In so doing, it might be important to hire counselors who are of the same ethnic background as the clients. In some cases, hiring Asian American counselors who have a different ethnic background may be inappropriate. For example, many traditional Korean Americans may not want to work with Japanese American counselors. In Chapter 2, I mentioned that Korean migration to Hawai'i ended abruptly in 1905 because the Japanese government forced the Korean king to stop the migration. The Japanese government took control of Korea, and in 1910 fully annexed the country to make it a part of Japan making Koreans second-class citizens. The annexation continued for 35 years until 1945 when Japan was defeated in World War II. This forceful take-over and the countless atrocities that were committed by the Japanese during these four decades continue to be a source of tension between many Koreans and Japanese. For a similar reason, other Asian Americans (e.g., Chinese, Filipino) may have trouble working with Japanese American counselors.

Third, the agencies' administrators should consider offering workshops to their staff members to educate them about counseling issues that are salient to Asian American clients. Perhaps multicultural counseling experts can be brought in to conduct these workshops and discuss ways in which staff members can be more culturally relevant, sensitive, and effective with these clients.

Fourth, when working with Asian American clients who are strongly enculturated, low acculturated, or both, counselors should consider discussing the issues of shame and embarrassment about seeking help. If it is suspected that the clients are embarrassed about their need for counseling, counselors should help the clients strategize effective ways to cope with these feelings. A secondary positive outcome of engaging in this process is that counselors may gain a great deal of information about clients' cultural norms and beliefs, which can subsequently benefit the counseling process. In addition to this direct intervention, another potentially useful strategy is to assign the clients to an ethnically similar counselor. Having a counselor with a similar ethnic background may lead the clients to have a greater appreciation for the normality and benefits of the help-seeking endeavor. However, it should be noted that some Asian American clients who are assigned to an ethnically similar counselor might feel an increased sense of shame and embarrassment because they may be sensitive to the fact that an in-group person will be learning about their problems. Therefore, the assignment of a counselor should be made in consultation with the client.

COUNSELING VIGNETTE

The Case of Yu-Wen

Yu-Wen is a 44-year-old Chinese American father of two children who has been married for 17 years. Yu-Wen came from China in the mid-1980s to become a graduate student at a university in the Midwest. He met his future wife, also from China, and got married. Initially, the couple intended to return to China after they finished their studies. However, when the U.S. government offered permanent residency as a result of the Tiananmen

Square massacre in 1989, they decided to remain in the United States. After finishing school, they moved to the West Coast and obtained entry-level managerial positions at small businesses in Chinatown. Although they are proficient in English and feel somewhat acculturated to the U.S. cultural norms, both Yu-Wen and his wife consider themselves to be traditional Chinese and have been trying to teach their children Chinese customs, traditions, and the Mandarin language. Also, their long-term goal is to eventually return to China where all of their relatives reside.

Recently, Yu-Wen, for no apparent reason, has been feeling down and depressed. He has increasingly felt very homesick and wanted to see his aging parents in China whom he has not seen in nearly ten years. He finally reports to his wife that he feels tired all the time and "just want to sleep all day." In fact, his wife has noticed that Yu-Wen has not been eating well and seems to have lost a few pounds. Yu-Wen, after much hesitation, also shares with his wife that he has had thoughts about ending his life by taking sleeping pills to just "get away from it all." Yu-Wen's wife, having seen a television commercial and a poster at her worksite about counseling being a good way to combat depression, encourages Yu-Wen to seek help from a professional counselor. However, Yu-Wen does not want to see a counselor because he is ashamed and embarrassed about not being able to control his feelings and overcome the negative thoughts. In addition, he does not see how sharing his personal issues with a total stranger can be helpful. Nonetheless, Yu-Wen's wife persists and finally convinces Yu-Wen to go the community counseling center located a couple of blocks away within Chinatown.

At the counseling center, Yu-Wen is given a choice between a Chinese American and a European American counselor. After some thought, Yu-Wen decides that he is more comfortable seeing the Chinese American counselor because the counselor might better understand his situation. During the first session, the counselor, noticing that Yu-Wen is nervous about sharing his feelings and skeptical about how helpful counseling will be, provides a detailed description of what counseling entails and how people can benefit from counseling. The counselor hopes that Yu-Wen will feel a bit more at ease once he knows what will occur in counseling and how it could help him. Also, the counselor talks to Yu-Wen about the fact that many people, particularly Asian Americans, tend to feel very hesitant about seeing a counselor because of the stigma involved in having a psychological difficulty. Here, the counselor hopes to normalize Yu-Wen's sense of embarrassment. The counselor also emphasizes that everything they discuss will be in strict confidence (within the bounds of legal limitations) and that Yu-Wen should take as much time as he needs to share his concerns. Feeling a little relieved, Yu-Wen then begins to talk about his difficulties ...

Based on this vignette, here are questions for further consideration:

If you were assigned to work with Yu-Wen, how might you conceptualize Yu-Wen's difficulties?

(continued)

To what extent would his migration background and living experiences in the United States influence this conceptualization?

What other information would you want to know about Yu-Wen to get a more comprehensive picture of his functioning?

What do you think about the counselor's intervention strategy during the first session?

What other things would you do to make Yu-Wen feel more comfortable in the session?

PSYCHOLOGICAL ASSESSMENT

Despite the general reluctance among many Asian Americans in seeking mental health services, there are Asian Americans who do enter counseling. However, many of these persons, like Yu-Wen, may enter with a great deal of skepticism and culture-related concerns, which, if left unattended, could lead to premature termination from counseling. Thus, it is important for counselors to conduct a thorough assessment of the client at the beginning of the counseling relationship.

As with any clients, counselors should assess a number of factors to obtain a good understanding about the clients' background and their reasons for seeking treatment. Some of the common areas of assessment are the nature, severity, and duration of the problem, and the ways in which the problem had been addressed in the past. In addition, it is very important for counselors to obtain information about the factors related to clients' cultural background, which could lead to more relevant and helpful counseling relationships and interventions. Such cultural factors for assessment include (a) acculturation, enculturation, and racial and ethnic identity statuses, (b) attitudes about counseling, (c) experiences with oppression, (d) beliefs about the locus of problem etiology and goal of counseling, (e) possible presence of culture-specific psychological disorders, (f) prevalence of psychosomatic symptoms, and (g) availability of indigenous sources of support.

Acculturation, Enculturation, and Racial and Ethnic Identity

When counselors assess Asian American clients, it is important to determine the degree to which they identify and adhere to the norms of the U.S. and Asian cultures. Recognizing the high degree of within-group variability among Asian Americans, assessing these constructs can help counselors avoid stereotyping the clients and understand the clients' unique cultural background. To this end, acculturation and enculturation can be assessed along the dimensions of cultural values, behaviors, knowledge, and identity. In addition, racial and ethnic identity can be assessed based on the Minority Identity Development. Asian Americans can be in one of the following five stages: Conformity, Dissonance, Resistance and Immersion, Introspection, and Synergistic Articulation and Awareness. The assessment of these constructs can also provide insights into the types of counseling interventions that may be effective with Asian American clients. Specifically, to the extent that Asian American clients adhere to the norms of and identify with the Asian culture, counselors may need to modify conventional modes of service for them to be effective. On other hand, to the extent that clients adhere to the norms of and identify with the U.S. culture, counselors may find that conventional modes of service can be effective.

Attitudes about Counseling

It is important for counselors to assess the client's attitude toward counseling. As discussed earlier, many Asian Americans tend to have negative attitudes about counseling and may be skeptical about the benefits from it. This is especially true if the clients are strongly enculturated, not acculturated, or both because they may have the additional burden of dealing with the shame and stigma associated with having psychological problems and the need to seek help from people outside of family and friends. Counselors should inquire with clients about their thoughts and feelings about entering counseling and the level of credibility they have about counseling. If the clients report a low level of credibility and less than positive attitudes, it would be important to address them, as was illustrated above in the case of Yu-Wen.

Experiences with Oppression

As described in Chapters 2 and 3, Asian Americans have been and continue to be victims of oppression in the United States. Consequently, Asian Americans remain vulnerable to negative mental health outcomes. Hence, it is important for counselors to assess the extent to which clients have been victimized by oppression and whether clients' presenting issues might be related to this oppression. In addition, all counselors need to remain open and aware of their own participation in creating oppressive situations. For example, as counselors, we are in a position of power to make a judgment about the level of pathology that is present in the clients. In this decision-making process, we should be careful not to impose our own worldview on the clients' situation, thereby incorrectly determining something that is culturally different as being culturally pathological.

Beliefs about the Locus of Problem Etiology and the Goal of Counseling

In conjunction with the information counselors have about their clients' acculturation, enculturation, and identity status, it may be useful also to assess their beliefs about the locus of problem etiology and their goal of counseling. The combination of information on acculturation, locus of problem etiology, and goal of counseling can be helpful in determining the most effective helping role that counselors can implement (Atkinson, Thompson, & Grant, 1993). According to Atkinson et al. (1993), the conventional helping roles in counseling and psychotherapy might be irrelevant to the life experiences and the unique needs of ethnic minorities, including Asian Americans, particularly if the clients are immigrants. These authors suggest including viable alternative helping roles that are distinct from the conventional counseling and psychotherapy roles. To this end, Atkinson et al. developed a model called the Three-Dimensional Model of Multicultural Counseling. This model includes the following three factors that can be used to determine the best helping role: acculturation, locus of problem etiology, and goal of counseling. As mentioned earlier, acculturation refers to the extent to which Asian American clients have adopted the cultural norms of the United States. Locus of problem etiology, according to Atkinson et al., refers to a continuum of problem causes that can range from external to internal. Problems that are imposed by the environment are considered as having an external origin, whereas problems arising from within a person are considered to have an internal cause. Problems with external etiology for Asian Americans often are a function of oppression, including discrimination and stereotyping. For problems with internal etiology, they include such things as mood swings, irrational fears, and weak impulse control. As for the goal of counseling, it can be portrayed as a continuum that ranges from preventive on one end to remedial on the other end.

According to the Three-Dimensional Model of Multicultural Counseling, the combinations of acculturation (high and low), locus of problem etiology (internal and external), and goal of counseling (prevention and remediation) leads to one of eight different helper roles: adviser, advocate, change agent, consultant, facilitator of indigenous support systems, facilitator of indigenous healing methods, counselor, and conventional psychotherapist. Later in this chapter, under the psychological treatment section, I will return to this model and describe the relations between these eight roles and the three factors that are assessed. I will also provide detailed descriptions of the eight roles and the research bearing on this model.

Presence of Culture-Specific Psychological Syndromes

An important area of assessment when working with Asian American clients is the possible presence of culture-specific psychological syndromes. This is particularly true if the clients are recent immigrants or who are highly enculturated. Given the diversity of ethnicities represented among Asian Americans, there are numerous culture-specific forms in which psychological problems may be manifested. A list of some culture-bound syndromes reflecting this variety and uniqueness within the Asian American population are presented in the *Diagnostic and Statistical Manual of Mental Disorders– Fourth Edition– Text Revision* (DSM-IV-TR; American Psychiatric Association, 2000); the DSM-IV-TR is a diagnostic tool commonly used by mental health professionals. Some of the ailments specific to Asians, and by extension Asian Americans, are: *amok* (a dissociative disorder; found in Malaysia, Laos, and the Philippines), *dhat* (anxiety and hypochondriasis disorder; found in India), *hwa-byung* ("anger syndrome"; found in Korea), *koro* (anxiety about the sex organ receding into the body and causing death; found in south and east Asia), *latah* (hypersensitivity to sudden fright; found in south and east Asia), *qi-gong psychotic reaction* (dissociative and paranoid symptoms; found in China), *shenjing shuairuo* (physical and mental fatigue symptoms; found in China), *shen-kui* (anxiety and panic symptoms; found in China and Taiwan), *shin-byung* (anxiety and somatic symptoms; found in Korea), and *taijin kyofusho* (similar to social phobia; found in Japan). It should be noted, however, that these syndromes might apply only to a limited number of Asian Americans who hold traditional Asian beliefs and worldviews.

Prevalence of Psychosomatic Symptoms

Many Asian American clients may somaticize their psychological distress (Nishio & Bilmes, 1987). This is especially true if the clients are traditional and strongly enculturated. When working with these clients, counselors might find it helpful to learn about the clients' beliefs about the effects of psychological problems on their physical health. Doing so could lead to a more holistic service. For example, if a counselor works with a Thai American client who is experiencing muscle pain and gastrointestinal problems as a result of stress from marital conflict, the counselor might collaborate with the client's physician to treat the physical symptoms while attending to the psychological problem. Certainly, treating the psychological ailments alone, or more typically the physical symptoms alone, may not lead to lasting relief from the psychological problems.

Availability of Indigenous Sources of Support

When counselors work with Asian American clients, it is also important to assess for possible sources of indigenous support systems. Especially for traditional Asian American clients, it may be helpful to receive support from the extended family and others in the community with whom they are familiar. In doing so, these clients can continue to maintain valuable interpersonal connections with important persons in their lives. In addition, these connections could help clients to not only feel supported by others but also to know that they still are integral members of the family and community. If Asian American clients who hold traditional values do not appear to have readily available sources of support from their families, counselors may do well to assess clients' openness to receiving support from community agencies or organizations serving Asian Americans (e.g., "mutual associations," temples, churches). For this to be possible, counselors should identify these agencies and organizations in their communities and maintain ongoing professional relationships with them. I realize that in some communities where the number of Asian Americans is small, finding these sources of support might be difficult. One way that this problem might be addressed would be to seek resources via the Internet. Perhaps an Internet search could yield sources in a nearby town of which the counselor was not aware.

| COUNSELING VIGNETTE | **The Case of Christine** |

Christine is a 30-year-old Vietnamese American lesbian woman from the Midwest who was adopted by a European American family in 1975 at the end of the Vietnam War. Christine's biological parents died during the war and she does not know whether she has any relatives in Vietnam. Growing up in the United States, Christine has benefited from a very loving family. For example, when she came out in her early 20s and revealed her lesbian identity, Christine's parents were very accepting and supportive. While she no longer lives with her parents, due to relocating to another Midwestern city for a job, she maintains close contact with her parents.

(continued)

Recently, Christine has become seriously concerned about her eating habits and body image. She often finds herself engaged in binge eating, which is usually followed by throwing up in the bathroom. Christine also has been obsessed about how she looks and has been working out at a gym for three hours a day for the last several weeks. Her goal is to tone her body to get to "the ideal shape." However, no matter how much she exercises, Christine is dissatisfied with how her body looks. Although these types of behavior began during the latter part of Christine's college years, the situation has worsened in the last year. Hence, she decides to go to a local mental health clinic to speak with a counselor.

The counselor begins the session by asking Christine to explain the concerns that has brought her in for counseling. After a thorough discussion about the nature, duration, and severity of the problem, the counselor asks about Christine's cultural background as a way to get to know her better. Christine shares that she is an adoptee from Vietnam but does not identify with the Vietnamese culture because she was raised by a European American family and in a community in the Midwest where there is not a sizable Vietnamese community. In addition, because she is unsure about how other Vietnamese Americans would feel about her sexual orientation, she has not made any efforts to make contact with other Vietnamese Americans. Although Christine is interested in learning more about the Vietnamese culture, she doesn't feel strongly about it. Christine also shares that she considers herself to be very acculturated to the dominant U.S. cultural norms and identifies herself as a member of this group, although she recognizes that she doesn't fit in with this group physically. Christine adds that she did experience some racism (e.g., called a "gook") when she was growing up because she looked "Asian," although this didn't bother her too much. Christine explains that she is mainly interested in working on the eating concerns and doesn't believe that her Vietnamese background has a significant role in it.

Based on this information, the counselor begins to employ conventional counseling theories and interventions to help Christine work through her disordered eating behavior. Interestingly, during a discussion about the possible sources of the ideal body image that she has been unsuccessfully trying to achieve, Christine mentions that perhaps she has been trying to "look European American" although she is a Vietnamese person in biological terms. The counselor adds that perhaps this "impossible task" might be a major source of her problem, which leads Christine to gain some important insights about herself …

Based on this vignette, here are questions for further consideration:

If you were assigned to work with Christine, how might you conceptualize her difficulties?

What other information would you want to know about Christine to get a more comprehensive picture of her functioning?

To what extent would her experiences as an adoptee might be contributing to her problem?

What do you think about the counselor's intervention strategy during the first session?

What do you think about the counselor's interpretation about why Christine might be experiencing her problems? How plausible is this hypothesis?

What other possible reasons are there that are related to Christine's difficulties?

What conventional strategies might you use to help Christine?

INDIGENOUS HEALING METHODS

Based on the results of a psychological assessment, counselors might consider taking one of two routes of treatment: (a) conventional counseling that integrates culturally relevant and sensitive interventions, and (b) referral to practitioners of indigenous healing methods. If a counselor determines that a traditional Asian American client would not do well with conventional forms of counseling, even with the augmentation of culturally relevant and sensitive interventions, the counselor might consider referring the client to practitioners of indigenous healing practices. Although some people may question the validity of indigenous treatment methods, there is clear documentation using Western research paradigms indicating that many Asian clients find these methods to be beneficial (e.g., Kendall, 1988; Meng, Luo, & Halbreich, 2002; Walters, 2001; Yi, 2000).

One type of indigenous healing methods that may be used involves *shamans* (Walsh, 1994). Shamans in anthropological terms are referred to as witches, witch doctors, wizards, medicine men or women, and sorcerers. It is believed that these individuals possess the power to enter an altered state of consciousness that leads them to cures for various psychological ailments. Shamans are individuals who were identified at birth to hold magical powers and who are then trained to become master shamans. Shamans are often called to service when displeased spirits who have possessed the individual are believed to cause the psychological ailments experienced by that person. It is believed that shamans have the power to exorcise the individuals of these spirits. There is some research evidence on the effectiveness of employing shamans for psychological problems among Asians (e.g., Kendall, 1988; Walters, 2001; Yi, 2000). For example, Walters (2001) describes how the use of rituals, metaphors, and other mythical devices used by shamans has led to strong therapeutic alliances in helping alcohol abusing individuals in a nomadic tribes.

Another type of indigenous healing is *ta'i chi ch'uan*, which originated in China and is used throughout East Asian countries. Ta'i chi ch'uan involves an exercise that has the purpose of inducing relaxation and meditation (Koh, 1981). It involves a complex pattern of slow movements of the arms and legs.

For example, one form of ta'i chi ch'uan includes a sequence of 25 complex movements that can be further isolated into 148 gestures (i.e., changes in arm or leg position). There has been some research on the effects of ta'i chi ch'uan on the mental health among its practitioners. A study reviewing the extant literature suggests that ta'i chi ch'uan enhances overall psychological well-being and mood (Sandlund & Norlander, 2000). However, it should be noted that it is not clear whether the positive effects of ta'i chi ch'uan are due solely to its relaxation and meditation components, or whether they are the consequence of various peripheral factors such as indulging in activities that are pleasurable and satisfying. Whatever the mechanism of action, it seems clear that ta'i chi ch'uan can have positive effects on the mental health of its practitioners.

A third type of indigenous healing method is acupuncture, which also originated in China and is used throughout East Asian countries. Acupuncture treatments are based on principles of Chinese medicine in which health and illness are viewed in terms of a balance between *yin* and *yang* forces (Meng et al., 2002). It is believed that the balance largely depends on the proper circulation of the vital energy *Qi* along energetic pathway. Acupuncture involves inserting small pins on specific points on the body to improve the proper circulation of this energy, which may be associated with psychological difficulties. It is believed that the pins help to restore curative energies that are spread to the rest of the body. Acupuncture has been used to treat depression, anxiety disorders, alcoholism, and substance abuse (Meng et al., 2002).

Although the use of indigenous healing methods may offer significant help to clients, counselors should not try to provide these indigenous healing practices unless they have been trained in these methods. To facilitate referral of clients to the practitioners of these types of services, counselors should work with local agencies and organizations serving Asian Americans to identify the practitioners of indigenous healing methods. Again, the use of the Internet could aid in this search.

COUNSELING VIGNETTE

The Case of Seon-chul

Seon-chul is a 63-year-old Korean American man who immigrated to an East Coast state last year. He came to join his daughter and her family after his wife passed away. Although he was hesitant about moving to another country, he felt it would be best for his extended family if he lived with his daughter. In addition, he could be with his grandchildren whom he has not been able to see regularly.

Although the time immediately after joining his daughter and her family was filled with joy and happiness, Seon-chul soon began to feel sad and lonely. He misses his life in Korea, particularly his wife with whom he had been married for 45 years. He also has had a very difficult time adjusting to the life in the United States. Because he does not speak English and does not know how to drive a car, he spends most days staying home and waiting for his grandchildren to return from school and his daughter and her husband to return from work. Consequently, he is not able to establish any friends with other Koreans in the area. When he does venture outside his home, he finds himself feeling very nervous and scared of the "strange neighborhood" where few people walk and there are so many cars.

After noticing that her father has been looking depressed, Seon-chul's daughter takes him to a Korean-speaking counselor in the nearby Korea-town. During the initial meeting, the counselor encourages Seon-chul to share his thoughts and feelings about living in the United States. Although Seon-chul hesitates to share at first, he finally opens up after the counselor explains to him that his family is very concerned and that to share would help the family as well. Seon-chul explains to the counselor that he very much misses his wife and wants to know that she was doing well in "the next world." He adds that if he was living in Korea he could go to a *mu-dang* (Korean shaman) who could communicate with his wife to let her know that he misses her and also to let him know how she is doing. Seon-chul also shares with the counselor that he has been having migraine headaches since he has moved to the United States, particularly when he ventures outside of home. Finally, Seon-chul reveals feeling very lonely and depressed during the past few months.

Based on all of this information, the counselor decides to treat Seon-chul using indigenous healing methods. Because the counselor does not have the training in these methods, the counselor seeks help from the Korean community. First, the counselor finds a *mu-dang* in Koreatown who eventually helps Seon-chul "communicate" with his wife. Second, the counselor finds an acupuncturist who treats Seon-chul for his headaches and depression. Third, the counselor helps Seon-chul enroll in a Korean senior citizens program, where he meets other Koreans elders and engages in enjoyable activities with them. Throughout this process, the counselor meets with Seon-chul weekly to see how all of these treatment interventions are progressing.

Based on this vignette, here are questions for further consideration:

If you were assigned to work with Seon-chul, how might you concep-tualize his difficulties? Would you differ from the counselor above?

What other information would you want to know about Seon-chul to get a more comprehensive picture of his functioning?

What do you think about the counselor's intervention strategies? How effective do they seem? Are there any other things you would do to help Seon-chul?

AREAS OF CONFLICT BETWEEN ASIAN AMERICANS' CULTURAL VALUES AND CONVENTIONAL APPROACHES TO PSYCHOLOGICAL TREATMENT

As described in Chapter 4, Asian American clients' adherence to Asian cultural values, a dimension of enculturation, can significantly affect counseling process and outcome (Kim, Atkinson, & Umemoto, 2001). Multicultural counseling scholars have suggested that the match or mismatch among client's cultural values, counselor's cultural values, and the values inherent in the counseling interventions determines counseling process effectiveness, and, distally, the counseling outcome (Atkinson, 2004; Sue & Sue, 2003). In other words, if counselors ignore the cultural values salient for Asian Americans and unknowingly promote ideals that conflict with these values, their interventions may not be as effective as expected.

Several examples can be generated in which a mismatch between conventional counseling approaches and Asian American clients' cultural values can lead to negative counseling process and outcome. Some counseling theories (e.g., Gestalt Theory) posit the notion that emotional expressions are beneficial and even curative to clients' problems. Imagine working with a Japanese American male client and strongly encouraging him to express the emotions he must have as he tells his story. If the client has a traditional value that being reticent is a sign of strength, not only will the counselor be asking the client to appear weak, the counselor may well embarrass the client with what sound like demands to lose control. The working alliance the counselor is trying to maintain may not be able to bear the resulting embarrassment.

Psychoanalytic theories suggest that it is important to explore the underlying unconscious dynamics that are causing clients' problems. These dynamics could often include unresolved issues with family members or other significant figures in one's early life. But if a counselor is working with a traditional Asian Indian who does not want to bring shame to his family, such exploration may be threatening and could leave him feeling disloyal to his family.

Many traditional Asian American clients tend to defer to authority figures and look toward counselors to provide guidance and possible solutions to their problems. If a traditional Laotian client is asked to treat the counselor as an equal, as is often called for by humanistic theories, this may lead the client to feel uncomfortable in the relationship.

Lastly, for Asian American clients who adhere to the value of being humble, having them openly describe their achievements and accomplishments as a way to dispute their negative self-concepts, as may be done in cognitive therapies, may be counterproductive and leave the clients feeling arrogant and offensive.

However, counselors should also keep in mind that some of the interactions between conventional counseling approaches and cultural values that are salient among traditional Asian Americans might lead to a positive counseling process and outcome. For example, the value of maintaining interpersonal harmony may lead a Thai American client to work just as hard as the counselor to form an effective working alliance, a key ingredient in humanistic counseling theories. In addition, the value of respecting and deferring to authority figures may allow counselors to have increased credibility, with which the counselors can increase their helpfulness with Asian American clients. The presence of these types of values among Asian American clients may enhance compliance with treatment strategies that are used by counselors.

In summary, to anticipate whether Asian cultural values will play helpful or impeding roles in counseling, counselors should identify the cultural values that are salient to their Asian American clients. To facilitate this process, counselors might present a list of Asian cultural values, as described in Chapter 4, to their clients and ask them to talk about the salience of these values to them. In doing so, counselors also may be able to gain useful information about the clients' background and presenting problems that may be related to their cultural values. Once important cultural values have been identified, counselors can formulate hypotheses about how these values may affect the counseling relationship and process and implement interventions that address these potentialities. In turn, these interventions may enhance the counseling process and help ensure a positive outcome.

COUNSELING VIGNETTE

The Case of Geeta

Geeta is a 28-year-old Asian Indian woman who recently entered the United States with a sponsorship from her relatives who immigrated soon after the passing of the 1965 Immigration Act. Because Geeta is from a lower-class group within India's caste system, there was little hope for educational or economic success for Geeta if she had remained in India. In addition, because her parents are poor and could not afford the dowry needed for her to get married, Geeta has remained a single woman, another fact that made immigration an attractive option for her. Unfortunately, however, because Geeta only has some high school education, she had to settle for working as a janitor at a large computer firm since arriving in the United States.

Recently, Geeta has been feeling very stressed with work. In particular, she has been experiencing many conflicts with her supervisor, who in Geeta's views has been treating her unfairly. Her supervisor has been assigning Geeta many more cleaning tasks than he has assigned to her male colleagues. Also, because Geeta speaks with an accent, her supervisor sometimes becomes irritated that he cannot readily understand her and needs to ask her to repeat herself. After a few weeks of this, Geeta decides to seek help from mental health counselors at the company's human resources department.

At the first session, the counselor asks Geeta to describe her reasons from coming in. After a thorough discussion about the dynamics between Geeta and her supervisor, the counselor, who has a psychoanalytic orientation, hypothesizes that Geeta's difficulties might be related to her perceptions of men as well as self-perception as a woman working in a male-dominated department. The counselor asks Geeta to talk more about her identity as a woman and views about women's role in society. During this discussion, the counselor asks Geeta to talk about her relationships with her family members and whether she has had any difficulties with males in her family. Geeta responds that her problem is with her supervisor and that it has nothing to do with her family. In addition, she mentions her desire to quit the job so that she can go to college, a wish that is not economically feasible for her. Nonetheless, the counselor continues to ask

(continued)

questions about Geeta's family dynamics when she was growing up. Feeling unhelped and frustrated, Geeta gets up and leaves the room ...

Based on this vignette, here are questions for further consideration:

If you were assigned to work with Geeta, how might you conceptualize her difficulties?

What other information would you want to know about Geeta to get a more comprehensive picture of her functioning?

What are some of the reasons that Geeta was feeling unhelped and frustrated? If you also have a psychoanalytic orientation, how might you tailor the counseling theory to better meet Geeta's problems?

What other counseling theories might better address Geeta's difficulties?

MODIFICATION OF CONVENTIONAL COUNSELING

If the psychological assessment results show that clients can benefit from conventional forms of counseling, care must be taken to augment the treatment with culturally relevant and sensitive strategies. There have been a number of research studies on counselor types and counseling interventions that may be effective with Asian American clients. In general, the findings suggest that Asian Americans favor ethnically similar counselors over ethnically dissimilar counselors (Atkinson, Maruyama, & Matsui, 1978; Atkinson & Matsushita, 1991; Atkinson, Poston, Furlong, & Mercado, 1989; Atkinson, Wampold, Lowe, Matthews, & Ahn, 1998) and counselors with similar attitudes, more education, older in age, and similar personality (Atkinson et al., 1989; Atkinson, Wampold, et al., 1998). Asian Americans also favor a logical, rational, and directive counseling style to a reflective, affective, and nondirective one (Atkinson et al., 1978), especially if the counselor is an Asian American (Atkinson & Matsushita, 1991). Asian Americans view culturally sensitive counselors as being more credible and culturally competent than less sensitive counselors (Gim, Atkinson, & Kim, 1991), and judge culturally responsive counselors as more credible than culturally neutral counselors (Zhang & Dixon, 2001). Asian Americans prefer counselors who express values that are similar to their values and who acknowledge racial differences when in a cross-racial client-counselor dyad (Li, Kim, & O'Brien, 2007). Research also suggests that bicultural Asian Americans perceive counselors as being more attractive than do Western-identified participants (Atkinson & Matsushita, 1991). Furthermore, a study by Merta, Ponterotto, and Brown (1992) suggests that acculturated Asian international student clients view authoritative peer counselors as being more credible than collaborative peer counselors.

Although these findings provide some insights into what might comprise effective counseling strategies when counselors work with Asian American clients, none of the studies, except for Merta et al. (1992), employed actual clients who were engaged in a realistic counseling situation. Instead, they utilized either surveys or audiovisual analogue designs, which rely on the ability of participants to accurately assume the role of clients based on reading counseling scripts, listening to audiotapes, or watching videotapes. As a result, one could question whether the findings are applicable to actual counseling sessions.

There have been some efforts to study counseling process using Asian American clients in actual counseling situations. The results in this research suggest that Asian American clients who have high adherence to Asian cultural values perceive counselors more positively than the clients who are low in adherence to Asian values (Kim, Li, & Liang, 2002; Kim, Ng, & Ahn, 2005). This is especially true if the counselors also are Asian Americans (Kim & Atkinson, 2002). These findings are consistent with the notion that the enculturated Asian Americans tend to defer to authority figures, such as professional counselors, and as a result, perceive them favorably (Gim et al., 1990; Atkinson et al., 1990).

In terms of counseling strategies, research suggests that Asian American clients favor the goal of looking for immediate resolution of the problem, rather the goal of exploring the problem to gain insight about its source (Kim et al., 2002). Research with actual clients also suggests that Asian Americans prefer a directive counseling style to a nondirective style (Li & Kim, 2004). In another study, Asian American clients rated counselors who disclosed personal information about successful strategies they themselves used in similar situations to be much more helpful than counselors who disclosed other types of personal information (Kim, Hill, et al., 2003). In addition, clients in this study also reported that counselors' disclosure about personal insights were helpful. Moreover, Asian American clients preferred counselors who tried to match the client's worldview in terms of a possible cause of the client's problem than counselors who did not match the worldview (Kim et al., 2005; Kim, Ng, & Ahn, 2009).

In general, many of these research findings are consistent with Sue and Zane's (1987) notion of "gift giving." The authors theorized that, for counselors to be perceived as culturally responsive and to reduce clients' premature termination, counselors should focus on helping clients to experience immediate and concrete psychological benefits of counseling in the initial sessions; they termed this strategy gift-giving. Examples of "gifts" are, in general, a resolution of a presenting problem, and, in particular, anxiety reduction, depression relief, cognitive clarity, normalization, and skills acquisition. Sue and Zane pointed out that ethnic minorities in general and Asian Americans in particular have the need to attain some type of meaningful gains early in counseling and "Gift giving demonstrates to clients the direct relationship between working in therapy and alleviation of problems" (p. 42). The current research literature on counseling Asian Americans provide support for these ideas and suggest that counselors may do well to provide immediate and concrete benefits to their Asian American clients at an early onset of counseling. In doing so, counselors may prevent these clients from premature termination and, ultimately, help the clients to resolve all of the presenting issues.

Another theoretical model that can be helpful when using the modified counseling approach is the Three-Dimensional Model of Multicultural

Counseling that was mentioned earlier. Recall that the model includes three factors (acculturation, locus of problem of etiology, and goal of counseling), a combination of which suggests the use of one of the following eight helper roles: adviser, advocate, change agent, consultant, facilitator of indigenous support systems, facilitator of indigenous healing methods, counselor, and conventional psychotherapist.

According to this model, if clients are low acculturated (e.g., a recent immigrant from Vietnam), have an external locus of problem of etiology (e.g., racism), and have a prevention goal, the suggested role is that of an *adviser*. In this role, a counselor would advise the Vietnamese American client about how to avoid a problem related to racism, which has occurred to other people in the past. If clients are low acculturated (e.g., a recent immigrant from Pakistan), have an internal locus of problem etiology (e.g., depression), and a prevention goal, the suggested role is that of *facilitator of indigenous support systems*. In this role, a counselor would seek additional sources of support for the Pakistani American client within the Pakistani American community. If clients are highly acculturated (e.g., a fifth-generation Japanese American), have an external etiology (racism), and have a prevention goal, the suggested role is that of a *consultant*. In this role, a counselor can help the Japanese American client learn the skills needed to interact successfully with the dominant society to avoid racism. If clients are highly acculturated (e.g., a fourth-generation Korean American), have an internal etiology (depression), and have a prevention goal, the suggested role is that of a *counselor*. This role involves providing counseling to the client to prevent future problems. Atkinson et al. proposed another role for alleviating existing problems (psychotherapist, which will be discussed later) and suggested that the difference is that the counselor role can be useful in teaching clients the necessary skills to avoid future problems.

Thus far, we have focused on preventing future problems. Now, let us look at the roles that are recommended by the Three-Dimensional Model for alleviating existing problems (Atkinson et al., 1993). If clients are low acculturated (e.g., a recent immigrant from Taiwan), have an external problem etiology (racism), and need remediation from current experiences with racism, the suggested role is that of an *advocate*. In this role, a counselor might speak on behalf of the Taiwanese client to confront and eliminate the sources of racism. For example, a Taiwanese child immigrant with normal intelligence who receives an inappropriate educational placement may benefit from a counselor advocating for placement in an appropriate bilingual setting. If clients are low acculturated (e.g., a recent immigrant from India), have an internal problem etiology (depression), and need remediation, the suggested role is *facilitator of indigenous healing methods*. Here, a counselor might refer the Asian Indian client to an indigenous healer, who may be perceived by the client as having a high degree of credibility. If clients are high acculturated (e.g., a fifth-generation Filipino American), have an external problem etiology (racism), and need to stop the current effects of racism, the suggested role is that of a *change agent*. In this role, a counselor would attempt to change the social environment that oppresses the Filipino American client and help the client identify both the sources of racism and methods of resolving the problem.

Finally, if clients are high acculturated (e.g., a fifth-generation Chinese American), have an internal problem etiology (depression), and need remediation from depression, the suggested role is that of a *conventional psychotherapist.* In this role, a counselor would provide psychotherapy to treat the depression experienced by the Chinese American client.

As can be seen, the Three-Dimensional Model of Multicultural Counseling can be very useful when working with Asian Americans. Indeed, a study by Atkinson, Kim, and Caldwell (1998) reported initial support for the roles specified by this model in the form of positive ratings by psychologists. In addition, this study found overwhelming support among Asian American college students for the consultant helping role when the presenting problem has an external etiology (e.g., racism) and the facilitator of indigenous support systems when the problem has an internal etiology (e.g., depression). It should be mentioned that although this model presents the eight roles as distinct ways to helping, counselors might use a combination of the roles based on the unique situation of each client. Hence, counselors should not feel limited by the distinctiveness of the eight roles, but rather be empowered to engage in helping activities suggested by all eight roles.

COUNSELING VIGNETTE

The Case of Maria

Maria is a 21-year-old Filipina American who entered the United States with her family when she was 12-years-old. Because she has been socialized into the Filipino culture before immigration and has learned the U.S. cultural norms, Maria considers herself to be a 1.5-generation American. In addition to cultural knowledge, Maria is proficient in both English and Tagalog, which allows her to be intimately involved in both the Filipino and the U.S. cultures and to maintain her strong bicultural status. Currently, Maria is in her third year at a local university where she is majoring in engineering. Although she has been able to maintain a decent grade-point average, her grades have not been stellar. In fact, Maria has not enjoyed any of her engineering courses, especially because there are no other Filipino American women, nor many women for that matter, in the major and she has experienced some racist and sexist remarks from non-Asian students. Hence, Maria has been completing the courses "just to get by". If she had her choice, Maria would change her major to psychology and eventually become a counselor. However, her parents feel very strongly about Maria becoming an engineer, which they believe can allow her to make a good living after she graduates. Trying to be a good daughter, Maria has not objected to her parents' wishes and has continued to remain in the major, while trying to cope with her unhappiness. However, she finally decides to see a counselor to discuss her concerns about her major and her unhappiness with it.

At her first session with a counselor, Maria says that she has never had counseling before and she is not sure how it can be beneficial to her.

(continued)

She adds that she wants to just try it because she has no other alternatives. After describing her unhappiness with her major, Maria says that she is a traditional Filipina and believes that it is important for her to fulfill her filial duties to her parents. As a result, she doesn't feel that changing her major is an option. The counselor responds by stating that she respects Maria's cultural values and agrees that changing her major doesn't seem to be a viable option for her. Making this statement allows the counselor to have a shared worldview with the client. At the same time, the counselor, using a directive style, suggests that she might consider applying for a volunteer position as a peer counselor at the counseling center. Doing so could allow Maria to do something that she enjoys while trying to figure out ways in which she can cope with her unhappiness in the major; this could serve as an immediate surface resolution to one of Maria's problems and a form of gift giving by the counselor. As the session concludes, Maria informs the counselor that the session was very helpful and that she is looking forward to returning for her next appointment.

After the session, the counselor also engages in the role of an advocate (as suggested in the Three Dimensional Model of Multicultural Counseling). With the permission of Maria, the counselor contacts the student advisor in the engineering department to inform the advisor about the racist and sexist comments that are being made by the students; during this advocacy, the counselor maintained strict confidentiality about her work with Maria. The counselor suggests to the advisor that cultural and gender sensitivity workshops be offered to the students in the major and the advisor thinks those are good ideas and agrees to do so ...

Based on this vignette, here are questions for further consideration:

If you were assigned to work with Maria, how might you conceptualize her difficulties?

What other information would you want to know about Christine to get a more comprehensive picture of her functioning?

What do you think about the counselor's intervention strategies with Maria?

What other strategies might you use to help Maria?

ADDITIONAL SOURCES OF MENTAL HEALTH SUPPORT

Whether counselors are using conventional counseling or facilitating the provision of indigenous healing methods with their Asian American clients, counselors might consider referring the Asian American clients for adjunctive support services to agencies or organizations serving Asian Americans. For example, it has been well-documented that Korean Americans are over-represented in churches in comparison to other ethnic groups and that they tend to seek support from church priests and other parishioners (Kim, 1977; Park, 1989). Hence, when working with a traditional Korean American client who is Christian, a counselor may do well to help establish a connection between the client and a local Korean church in the community. Similarly, a counselor might refer traditional Vietnamese American Buddhist client to temples in which priests can provide supportive services. One inherent benefit of utilizing existing sources of support found within the ethnic communities is that service providers may be able to speak the native languages of the clients. However, before making any referral recommendations, it is important for counselors to know what roles churches or temples have played in the clients' lives in the past and determine how helpful the current referral might be. Also, although using culture-based sources of support may be useful, care should be taken so that the clients will not experience shame and embarrassment. This may occur if other members of the community learn that these individuals suffer from psychological difficulties. To avoid such situations, counselors should work closely with their clients to identify support sources with which the clients feel comfortable.

There have been a couple of research studies that support the use the community sources of support. As mentioned previously, Atkinson, Kim, and Caldwell (1998) found that Asian American college students endorsed the use of indigenous support systems when Asian American clients experience problems that are internal in nature (e.g., depression). Indigenous support systems include culturally compatible religious or community centers designed to serve Asian American clients. In a study utilizing a qualitative method, Kim et al. (2003) found that, while Asian American participants had negative attitudes toward seeking help from counselors and psychologists, participants were very open to seeking emotional support from community organizations, such as churches. To be able to make these referrals, it is critical, as noted previously, for counselors to be in contact with ethnic organizations in the communities and be aware of the types of resources that are available.

COUNSELING VIGNETTE

The Case of James

James is a 17-year-old biracial Asian and European American whose ancestors from Japan arrived in the United States in the early 1900s and ancestors from Ireland and Italy arrived in the mid-1800s. He considers himself to be a fifth-generation American on his Japanese side and sixth-generation American on his Irish and Italian side. James is well acculturated to U.S. cultural norms and is somewhat familiar with his Japanese, Irish, and Italian backgrounds. If asked what ethnic background he identifies to a greater extent with, he indicates that this is a very difficult question because he identifies with all three ethnic backgrounds as well as the "U.S. identity." He feels like he is a "mixed breed" and it would be very difficult for him to choose one background over another. However, he sometimes feels like he doesn't belong to any of these groups. For example, at his school, he is not treated as an Italian person by other Italian Americans because he does not look Italian. Similarly, other Japanese and Irish Americans also treat him differently. When this occurs, he struggles to maintain a sense of ethnic identity for himself, which has not been easy. Currently,

(continued)

James wants to learn more about the traditional Japanese, Irish, and Italian customs and traditions and perhaps major in ethnic studies when he goes to college. His goal is to get a better sense of the experiences of biracial and multiracial persons (like himself) in the United States.

James, as a senior in high school, has been experiencing a lot of stress trying to complete his courses while applying to a number of colleges. His college entrance examination scores are good but not great so he has concerns about whether he will be admitted to his top choice school that has a fabulous ethnic studies program. After having been unable to sleep and eat as a result of this stress, James finally seeks the help of his school counselor.

During the sessions, the counselor learns about James's concerns regarding college and how he feels pressured to get into the college with the top ethnic studies program. The counselor also learns that despite these worries, there isn't anything James can do but to wait for the decision. Hence, the counselor works with James to discuss the implications for a range of possible outcomes, one of which is that he is not accepted into his top school but to a small local college. In discussing the pros and cons of attending the local college, James mentions that he can be close to the nearby Japantown and Little Italy where he can visit regularly to learn more about two of his cultural heritages. Based on this idea, the counselor suggests that James might volunteer at the community center in either Japantown or Little Italy where he can participate in cultural activities. James agrees to this idea and becomes a volunteer at a center.

Later that school year, James learns that he did not get into his first choice school but only to the local college. While attending the local school, James continues to work at the community center and gain valuable experience. The following year, James is able to transfer to his top choice school with the help from the director of the community center who wrote him an excellent letter of recommendation.

Based on this vignette, here are questions for further consideration:

If you were assigned to work with James, how might you conceptualize his difficulties?

What other information would you want to know about James to get a more comprehensive picture of his functioning?

What do you think about the counselor's intervention strategies with James?

What other strategies might you use to help James?

SUMMARY AND RECOMMENDATIONS

Based on the information provided above, the following treatment recommendations can be made. To meet the mental health needs of Asian Americans and increase their utilization of counseling services, counselors might consider conducting outreach services. In addition, counselors might attend to and address feelings of shame and embarrassment by Asian Americans who enter counseling. During an initial assessment of clients, counselors could assess their levels of acculturation and enculturation and the stage of racial and ethnic identity in order to determine the degree to which conventional modes of counseling will be relevant and effective with the clients. If the clients are acculturated and identify with the U.S. culture, conventional modes of treatment may be effective. On the other hand, if clients are enculturated and identify with the Asian culture, conventional modes of treatment need to be altered to infuse increased levels of cultural relevance and sensitivity. Also, counselors might try to gather information about the clients' attitudes regarding counseling, their experiences with oppression (discrimination and prejudice), their beliefs about the source of the problem, their goal of counseling, possible sources of culture-specific psychological disorders, signs of psychosomatic symptoms, and additional sources of mental health support. These types of information may provide counselors with insights about the level of credibility ascribed to counselors by the clients, cross-cultural relationships that may be associated with the presenting problems, and important and potentially useful sources of emotional support.

After assessing clients' acculturation levels locus of problem etiologies and goals of counseling, counselors may refer to Atkinson et al.'s (1993) Three Dimensional Model for Counseling Racial/Ethnic Minorities to determine appropriate helper roles for their Asian American clients. Also, for traditional Asian American clients (i.e., high enculturation, low acculturation, or both), especially those who are mistrustful of conventional treatment providers, counselors might consider making referrals to cultural resources within the community, practitioners of indigenous healing methods, or both. When counseling traditional Asian American clients, counselors may be more effective when counselors are ethnically similar. Hence, counselors might make an effort to assign Asian American clients to ethnically similar counselors. In addition, counselors may be effective if they use a directive, logical, rational counseling style. Counselors also should try to focus on providing immediate and concrete benefits of counseling, especially during the early stages of the counseling relationship. As mentioned earlier, "gift giving" (Sue & Zane, 1987) can be an important mechanism by which counselors can ensure that clients will return for subsequent sessions. The use of gift giving to clients also may increase the likelihood that clients comply with subsequent treatment interventions. In addition to these strategies, counselors, especially if they are not of Asian American background, may enhance their credibility with Asian American clients by acknowledging the different cultural background and that this difference may impact the counseling relationship and effectiveness. Counselors also may enhance their credibility by attending to cultural influences on the presenting issues. Counselors also might inform the clients that they are open to learning as much as possible about the clients' cultural background because doing so can increase their helpfulness to the clients. Throughout the counseling process, counselors might inquire with the clients about the cultural appropriateness of their interventions and make adjustments based on client feedback.

Finally, I would like to wish you much success on your journey toward becoming a culturally relevant, sensitive, and effective counselor with Asian American clients! Thank you for allowing me to accompany you in these first steps of your journey.

A RESOURCE LIST FOR FURTHER READING

Below is a list of resources to learn more about counseling Asian American clients.

Atkinson, D. R. (2004). *Counseling American minorities* (6th ed.). Boston: McGraw-Hill.

Bernal, G., Trimble, J. E., Burlew, A. K., & Leong, F. T. L. (2003). *Handbook of racial and ethnic minority psychology.* Thousand Oaks, CA: Sage Publications.

Constantine, M. G. (Ed.). (2007). *Clinical practice with people of color: A guide to becoming culturally competent.* New York: Teachers College Press.

Hall, G. C. N., & Barongan, C. (2002). *Multicultural psychology.* Upper Saddle River, NJ: Prentice-Hall.

Hall, G. C. N., & Okazaki, S. (2002). *Asian American psychology: The science of lives in context.* Washington, D.C.: American Psychological Association.

Hampton, N. Z., & Chang, V. (2002). *Quality of life as defined by Chinese Americans with disabilities: Implications for rehabilitation counseling.* Boston: Institute of Asian American Studies, University of Massachusetts-Boston.

Hong, G. K., & Ham, M. D. (2001). *Psychotherapy and counseling for Asian American clients: A practical guide.* Thousand Oaks, CA: Sage.

Kodama, C. M., McEwen, M. K., Alvarez, A. N., Liang, C., & Lee, S., (Eds.). (2002). *Working with Asian American college students: New directions for student services.* San Francisco: Jossey Bass.

Leong, F. T. L., Inman, A. G., Ebreo, A., Yang, L. H., Kinoshita, L., & Fu, M. (Eds.). (2007). *Handbook of Asian American Psychology* (2nd ed.). Thousand Oaks, CA: Sage.

Mio, J. S., & Iwamasa, G. Y. (Eds.). (2003). *Culturally diverse mental health: The challenge of research and resistance.* New York: Brunner-Routledge.

Nam, V. (Ed.). (2001). *YELL-Oh Girls! Emerging voices explore culture, identity, and growing up Asian American.* New York: HarperCollins Publishers.

Smith, T. B. (Ed.). (2004). *Practicing multiculturalism: Affirming diversity in counseling and psychology.* Boston: Allyn and Bacon.

Sue, D. W. (2003). *Overcoming our racism: The journey to liberation.* San Francisco: Jossey-Bass

Sue, D. W. & Sue, D. (2003). *Counseling the culturally diverse: Theory and practice.* (4th ed.). New York: Houghton Mifflin.

Tewari, N. & Alvarez, A. N. (Eds.). (2009). *Asian American psychology: Current perspectives.* New York: Taylor & Francis Group.

Trinh, N., Rho, Y. C., Lu, F. G., & Sanders, K. M. (Eds.). (2009). *Handbook of mental health and acculturation in Asian American families.* New York: Humana Press.

Uba, L. (2002). *A postmodern psychology of Asian Americans: Creating knowledge of a racial minority.* Albany, NY: State University of New York Press.

Vacc, N. A., DeVaney, S. B., & Brendel, J. M. (Eds.). (2003). *Counseling multicultural and diverse populations: Strategies for practitioners.* New York: Brunner-Routledge.

REFERENCES

Ahn, A. J., Kim, B. S. K., & Park, Y. S. (2008). Asian cultural values gap, cognitive flexibility, coping strategies, and parent-child conflicts among Korean Americans. *Cultural Diversity and Ethnic Minority Psychology, 14,* 353–363.

American Psychiatric Association. (2000). *Diagnostic and statistical manual of mental disorders* (4th ed.). Washington, DC: Author.

Asamen, J. K., & Berry, G. L. (1987). Self-concept, alienation, and perceived prejudice: Implications for counseling Asian Americans. *Journal of Multicultural Counseling and Development, 15,* 146–160.

Atkinson, D. R., & Gim, R. H. (1989). Asian-American cultural identity and attitudes toward mental health services. *Journal of Counseling Psychology, 36,* 209–212.

Atkinson, D. R., Kim, B. S. K., & Caldwell, R. (1998). Ratings of helper roles by multicultural psychologists and Asian American students: Initial support for the three-dimensional model of multicultural counseling. *Journal of Counseling Psychology, 45,* 414–423.

Atkinson, D. R., Lowe, S. M., & Matthews, L. (1995). Asian-American acculturation, gender, and willingness to seek counseling. *Journal of Multicultural Counseling and Development, 23,* 130–138.

Atkinson, D. R., Maruyama, M., & Matsui, S. (1978). The effects of counselor race and counseling approach on Asian Americans' perceptions of counselor credibility and utility. *Journal of Counseling Psychology, 25,* 76–83.

Atkinson, D. R., & Matsushita, Y. J. (1991). Japanese-American acculturation, counseling style, counselor ethnicity, and perceived counselor credibility. *Journal of Counseling Psychology, 38,* 473–478.

Atkinson, D. R. (2004). *Counseling American minorities* (6th ed.). Boston, MA: McGraw-Hill.

Atkinson, D. R., Poston, W. C., Furlong, M. J., & Mercado, P. (1989). Ethnic group preferences for counselor characteristics. *Journal of Counseling Psychology, 36,* 68–72.

Atkinson, D. R., Thompson, C. E., & Grant, S. K. (1993). A three-dimensional model for counseling racial/ethnic minorities. *The Counseling Psychologist, 21,* 257–277.

Atkinson, D. R., Wampold, B. E., Lowe, S. M., Matthews, L., & Ahn, H. (1998). Asian American preference for counselor characteristics: Application of the Bradley-Terry-Luce model to paired comparison data. *The Counseling Psychologist, 26,* 101–123.

Atkinson, D. R., Whiteley, S., & Gim, R. H. (1990). Asian-American acculturation preferences for help providers. *Journal of College Student Development, 31,* 155–161.

Barnes, J. S., & Bennett, C. E. (2002). *The Asian population: 2000.* Retrieved August 27, 2009, from http://www.census.gov/prod/2002pubs/c2kbr01-16.pdf.

Bauman, K. J., & Graf, N. L. (2003). Educational attainment: 2000. Retrieved August 27, 2009, from http://www.census.gov/prod/2003pubs/c2kbr-24.pdf.

Berry, J. W. (1980). Acculturation as varieties of adaptation. In A. M. Padilla (Ed.), *Acculturation: Theory, models, and some new findings* (pp. 9–25). Boulder, CO: Westview Press.

Berry, J. W. (1990). Psychology of acculturation: Understanding individuals moving between cultures. In R. W. Brislin (Ed.), *Applied cross-cultural psychology* (pp. 232–253). Newbury Park, CA: Sage Publications.

Berry, J. W. (1994). Acculturation and psychological adaptation: An overview. In A. Bouvy, F. J. R. van de Vijver, P. Boski, & P. Schmitz (Eds.), *Journeys into cross-cultural psychology* (pp. 129–141). Amsterdam, Holland: Swets & Zeitlinger.

Berry, J. W., & Annis, R. C. (1974). Acculturative stress: The role of ecology, culture and differentiation. *Journal of Cross-Cultural Psychology, 5,* 382–406.

Berry, J. W., & Kim, U. (1988). Acculturation and mental health. In P. R. Dasen, J. W. Berry, & N. Sartorius (Eds.), *Health and cross-cultural psychology: Toward applications* (pp. 207–236). Newbury Park, CA: Sage Publications.

Berry, J. W., Kim, U., Power, S., Young, M., & Bajaki, M. (1989). Acculturation attitudes in plural societies. *Applied Psychology: An International Review, 38,* 185–206.

Berry, J. W., Trimble, J. E., & Olmeda, E. L. (1986). Assessment of acculturation. In W. J. Lonner & J. W. Berry (Eds.), *Field methods in cross-cultural research* (pp. 291–324). Newbury Park, CA: Sage Publications.

Broman, C. L. (1997). Race-related factors in life satisfaction among African Americans. *Journal of Black Psychology, 23,* 36–49.

Caplan, N., Whitmore, J. K., & Choy, M. H. (1989). *The boat people and achievement in America: A study of family life, hard work, and cultural values.* Ann Arbor: The University of Michigan Press.

Chan, S. (1991). *Asian Americans: An interpretive history.* Boston: Twayne Publishers.

Chan, S. (1994). *Hmong means free: Life in Laos and America.* Philadelphia: Temple University Press.

Chen, P. N. (1982). Eroding filial piety and its implications for social work practice. *Journal of Sociology and Social Welfare, 9,* 511–523.

Chung, R. H. G. (2001). Gender, ethnicity, and acculturation in intergenerational conflict of Asian American college students. *Cultural Diversity & Ethnic Minority Psychology, 7,* 376–386.

Committee of 100. (2001). *American attitudes toward Chinese Americans and Asian Americans.* New York: Author.

Crystal, D. (1989). Asian Americans and the myth of the model minority. *Social Casework, 70,* 405–413.

Cuellar, I., Arnold, B., & Maldonado, R. (1995). Acculturation rating scale for Mexican Americans-II: A revision of the original ARSMA scale. *Hispanic Journal of Behavioral Sciences, 17,* 275–304.

DeNavas-Walt, C., Proctor, B. D., & Smith, J. C. (2008). Income, poverty, and health insurance coverage in the United States: 2007. Retrieved August 28, 2009, from http://www.census.gov/prod/2008pubs/p60-235.pdf.

Espiritu, Y. L. (1995). *Filipino American lives.* Philadelphia: Temple University Press.

Etcheson, C. (1984). *The rise and demise of Democratic Kampuchea.* Boulder, CO: Westview Press.

Fang, C. Y., & Myers, H. F. (2001). The effects of racial stressors and hostility on cardiovascular reactivity in African American and Caucasian men. *Health Psychology, 20,* 64–70.

Fernandez, M. S. (1988). Issues in counseling Southeast-Asian students. *Journal of Multicultural Counseling and Development, 16,* 1157–166.

Fischer, A. R., & Shaw, C. M. (1999). African Americans' mental health and perceptions of racist discrimination: The moderating effects of racial socialization experiences and self-esteem. *Journal of Counseling Psychology, 46,* 395–407.

Freeman, J. M. (1995). *Changing identities: Vietnamese Americans, 1975–1995.* Boston: Allyn and Bacon.

Gibson, C., & Jung, K. (2002). *Historical census statistics on population totals by race, 1790 to 1990, and by Hispanic origin, 1970 to 1990, for the United States, regions, divisions, and states.* Retrieved August 27, 2009, from http://www.census.gov/population/www/documentation/twps0056.html.

Gim, R. H., Atkinson, D. R., & Kim, S. J. (1991). Asian-American acculturation, counselor ethnicity and cultural sensitivity, and ratings of counselors. *Journal of Counseling Psychology, 38,* 57–62.

Gim, R. H., Atkinson, D. R., & Whiteley, S. (1990). Asian-American acculturation, severity of concerns, and willingness to see a counselor. *Journal of Counseling Psychology, 37,* 281–285.

Graves, T. D. (1967). Psychological acculturation in a tri-ethnic community. *Southwestern Journal of Anthropology, 23,* 337–350.

Greenwald, A. G., & Banaji, M. R. (1995). Implicit social cognition: Attitudes, self-esteem, and stereotypes. *Psychological Review, 102,* 4–27.

Gudykunst, W. B. (2001). *Asian American ethnicity and communication.* Thousand Oaks, CA: Sage.

Herskovits, M. J. (1948). *Man and his works: The science of cultural anthropology.* New York: Knopf.

Ho, M. K. (1987). *Family therapy with ethnic minorities.* Newbury Park, CA: Sage Publications, Inc.

Hsia, J., & Peng, S. S. (1998). Academic achievement and performance. In L. C. Lee & N. W. S. Zane (Eds.), *Handbook of Asian American psychology* (pp. 325–358). Thousand Oaks, CA: Sage.

Hune, S., & Chan, K. S. (1997). Special focus: Asian Pacific American demographic and educational trends. In D. J. Carter & R. Wilson (Eds.), *Minorities in higher education: Fifteenth annual status report* (pp. 39–67). Washington, D.C.: American Council on Education.

Hwang, W. (2007). Acculturative family distancing: Theory, research, and clinical practice. *Psychotherapy Theory, Research, Practice, Training, 43,* 397–409.

Jensen, J. (1988). *Passage from India: Asian Indian immigrants in North America.* New Haven, CT: Yale University Press.

Kaneshige, E. (1973). Cultural factors in group counseling and interaction. *Personnel and Guidance Journal, 51,* 407–412.

Kendall, L. (1988). Healing thyself: A Korean shaman's afflictions. *Social Science and Medicine, 27,* 445–450.

Kim, B. C. (1973). Asian Americans: No model minority. *Social Work, 18,* 44–53.

Kim, B. S. K. (2007). Adherence to Asian and European American cultural values and attitudes toward seeking professional psychological help among Asian American college students. *Journal of Counseling Psychology, 54,* 474–480.

Kim, B. S. K., & Abreu, J. M. (2001). Acculturation measurement: Theory, current instruments, and future directions. In J. G. Ponterotto, J. M. Casas, L. A. Suzuki, & C. M. Alexander (Eds.), *Handbook of multicultural counseling* (2nd ed., pp. 394–424). Thousand Oaks, CA: Sage.

Kim, B. S. K., & Atkinson, D. R. (2002). Asian American client adherence to Asian cultural values, counselor expression of cultural values, counselor ethnicity, and career counseling process. *Journal of Counseling Psychology, 49,* 3–13.

Kim, B. S. K., Atkinson, D. R., & Umemoto, D. (2001). Asian cultural values and the counseling process: Current knowledge and directions for future research. *The Counseling Psychologist, 29,* 570–603.

Kim, B. S. K., Atkinson, D. R., & Yang, P. H. (1999). The Asian values scale: Development, factor analysis, validation, and reliability. *Journal of Counseling Psychology, 46,* 342–352.

Kim, B. S. K., Brenner, B. R., Liang, C. T. H., & Asay, P. A. (2003). A qualitative study of adaptation experiences of 1.5-generation Asian Americans. *Cultural Diversity and Ethnic Minority Psychology, 9,* 156–170.

Kim, B. S. K., D'Andrea, M., Sahu, P., & Gaughen, K. (1998). A multicultural study of university students' knowledge of and attitudes toward homosexuality. *Journal of Humanistic Education and Development, 36,* 171–182.

Kim, B. S. K., Hill, C. E., Gelso, C. J., Goates, M. K., Asay, P. A., & Harbin, J. M. (2003). Counselor self-disclosure, east Asian American client adherence to Asian cultural values, and counseling process. *Journal of Counseling Psychology, 50,* 324–332.

Kim, B. S. K., Li, L. C., & Liang, C. T. H. (2002). Effects of Asian American client adherence to Asian cultural values, session goal, and counselor emphasis of client expression on career counseling process. *Journal of Counseling Psychology, 49,* 342–354.

Kim, B. S. K., Ng, G. F., & Ahn, A. J. (2005). Effects of client expectation for counseling success, client-counselor worldview match, and client adherence to Asian and European American cultural values on counseling process with Asian Americans. *Journal of Counseling Psychology, 52,* 67–76.

Kim, B. S. K., Ng, G. F., & Ahn, A. J. (2009). Client adherence to Asian cultural values, common factors in counseling, and session outcome with Asian American clients at a university counseling center. *Journal of Counseling and Development, 87,* 131–142.

Kim, B. S. K., & Omizo, M. M. (2003). Asian cultural values, attitudes toward seeking professional psychological help, and willingness to see a counselor. *The Counseling Psychologist, 31,* 343–361.

Kim, B. S. K., & Omizo, M. M. (2005). Asian and European American cultural values, collective self-esteem, acculturative stress, cognitive flexibility, and general self-efficacy among Asian American college students. *Journal of Counseling Psychology, 52,* 412–419.

Kim, B. S. K., & Omizo, M. M. (2006). Behavioral acculturation and enculturation and psychological functioning among Asian American college students. *Cultural Diversity and Ethnic Minority Psychology, 12,* 245–258.

Kim, B. S. K., & Omizo, M. M. (2009). *Behavioral enculturation and acculturation, psychological functioning, and help-seeking attitudes among Asian American adolescents.* Manuscript submitted for publication

Kim, B. S. K., Yang, P. H., Atkinson, D. R., Wolfe, M. M., & Hong, S. (2001). Cultural value similarities and differences among Asian American ethnic groups. *Cultural Diversity and Ethnic Minority Psychology, 7,* 343–361.

Kim, H. (1977). The history and role of the church in the Korean American community. In H. Kim (Ed.), *The Korean Diaspora: Historical and sociological studies of Korean immigration and assimilation in North America* (pp. 47–63). Santa Barbara: ABC Clio, Inc.

Kim, I. (1981). *New urban immigrants: The Korean community in New York.* Princeton, New York: Princeton University Press

Kincaid, D. L., & Yum, J. O. (1987). A comparative study of Korean, Filipino, and Samoan immigrants in Hawaii: Socioeconomic consequences. *Human Organization, 46,* 70–77.

Kinzie, J. D. & Tseng, W. S. (1978). Cultural aspects of psychiatric clinic utilization: A cross-cultural study in Hawaii. *International Journal of Social Psychiatry, 24,* 177–188.

Kitano, H. H. L., & Matsushima, N. (1981). Counseling Asian Americans. In P. B. Pedersen, J. G. Draguns, W. J. Lonner, & J. E. Trimble (Eds.), *Counseling across cultures*

(2nd ed., pp. 163–180). Honolulu, HI: University of Hawaii Press.

Kluckhohn, C. (1951). The study of culture. In D. Lerner & H. D. Lasswell (Eds.), *The policy sciences* (pp. 86–101). Stanford, CA: Stanford University Press.

Koh, T. C. (1981). Tai chi chuan. *American Journal of Chinese Medicine, 9,* 15–22.

LaFromboise, T., Coleman, H. L K., & Gerton, J. (1993). Psychological impact of biculturalism: Evidence and theory. *Psychological Bulletin, 114,* 395–412.

Leong, F. T. L. (1994). Asian Americans' differential patterns of utilization of inpatient and outpatient public mental health services in Hawaii. *Journal of Community Psychology, 22,* 82–96.

Leong, F. T. L., & Serafica, F. C. (1995). Career development of Asian Americans: A research area in need of a good theory. In F. T. L. Leong (Ed.), *Career development and vocational behavior of racial and ethnic minorities* (pp. 67–102). Mahwah, NJ: Lawrence Erlbaum Associates, Inc.

Leong, F. T. L., Wagner, N. S., & Tata, S. P. (1995). Racial and ethnic variations in help-seeking attitudes. In J. G. Ponterotto, J. M. Casas, L. A. Suzuki, & C. M. Alexander (Eds.). *Handbook of multicultural counseling* (pp. 415–438). Thousand Oaks, CA: Sage Publications.

Lessinger, J. (1995). *From the Ganges to the Hudson: Indian immigrants in New York City.* Boston: Allyn and Bacon.

Li, L. C., & Kim, B. S. K. (2004). Effects of counseling style and client Adherence to Asian cultural values on counseling process with Asian American college students. *Journal of Counseling Psychology, 51,* 158–167.

Li, L. C., Kim, B. S. K., & O'Brien, K. M. (2007). An analogue study of the effects of Asian cultural values and counselor multicultural competence on counseling process. *Psychotherapy Theory, Research, Practice, Training, 44,* 90–95.

Liang, C. T. H., Li, L. C., & Kim, B. S. K. (2004). The Asian American Racism-Related Stress Inventory: Development, factor analysis, reliability, and validity. *Journal of*

Counseling Psychology, 51, 103–114.

Mendoza, R. H. (1984). Acculturation and sociocultural variability. In J. L. Martinez Jr. & R. H. Mendoza (Eds.), *Chicano Psychology* (2nd ed., pp. 61–74). New York: Academic Press, Inc.

Mendoza, R. H. (1989). An empirical scale to measure type and degree of acculturation in Mexican-American adolescents and adults. *Journal of Cross-Cultural Psychology, 20,* 372–385.

Meng, F., Luo, H., & Halbreich, U. (2002). Concepts, techniques, and clinical applications of acupuncture. *Psychiatric Annals, 32,* 45–49.

Merta, R. J., Ponterotto, J. G., & Brown, R. D. (1992). Comparing the effectiveness of two directive styles in the academic counseling of foreign students. *Journal of Counseling Psychology, 39,* 214–218.

Miller, M. J. (2007). A bilinear multi-dimensional measurement model of Asian American acculturation and enculturation: Implications for counseling interventions, *Journal of Counseling Psychology, 54,* 118–131.

Min, P. G. (1996). *Caught in the middle: Korean communities in New York and Los Angeles.* Berkeley: University of California Press.

Morrow, R. D. (1989). Southeast-Asian parental involvement: Can it be a reality? *Elementary School Guidance and Counseling, 23,* 289–297.

Moyerman, D. R., & Forman, B. D. (1992). Acculturation and adjustment: A meta-analytic study. *Hispanic Journal of Behavioral Sciences, 14,* 163–200.

National Asian Pacific American Legal Consortium (1999). *Audit of violence against Asian Pacific Americans: Challenging the invisibility of hate.* Washington, D. C.: Author.

National Asian Pacific American Legal Consortium (2001). *Backlash: When America turned on its own.* Washington, D.C.: Author.

Nicassio, P. M., Solomon, G. S., Guest, S. S., & McCullough, J. E. (1986). Emigration stress and language proficiency as correlates of depression in a sample of Southeast Asian refugees. *International Journal of Social Psychiatry, 32,* 22–28.

Nishio, K., & Bilmes, M. (1987). Psychotherapy with Southeast Asian American clients. *Professional Psychology: Research and Practice, 18,* 342–346.

Nwadiora, E., & McAdoo, H. (1996). Acculturative stress among Amerasian refugees: Gender and racial differences. *Adolescence, 31,* 477–487.

Omizo, M. M., Kim, B. S. K., & Abel, N. R. (2008). Asian and European American cultural values, bicultural competence, and attitudes toward seeking professional psychological help among Asian American adolescents. *Journal of Multicultural Counseling and Development, 36,* 15–28.

Ong, P., Bonacich, E. & Cheng, L. (1994). *The new Asian immigration in Los Angeles and global restructuring.* Philadelphia, PA: Temple University Press.

Ong, P., & Liu, J. M. (1994). U.S. immigration policies and Asian migration. In P. Ong, Bonacich, E., & Cheng, L. (Eds.), *The new Asian immigration in Los Angeles and global restructuring* (pp. 45–73). Philadelphia: Temple University Press.

Padilla, A. M. (1980). The role of cultural awareness and ethnic loyalty in acculturation. In A. M. Padilla (Ed.), *Acculturation: Theory, models, and some new findings* (pp. 47–84). Boulder, CO: Westview Press, Inc.

Park, K. (1989). "Born again": What does it mean to Korean-Americans in New York City? *Journal of Ritual Studies, 3/2,* 287–301.

Park, Y. S., & Kim, B. S. K. (2008). Asian and European American cultural values and communication styles among Asian American and European American college students. *Cultural Diversity and Ethnic Minority Psychology, 14,* 47–56.

Patterson, W. (1988). *The Korean frontiers in American: Immigration to Hawaii, 1896–1910.* Honolulu: University of Hawaii Press.

Peterson, W. (1966, January 9). Success story: Japanese American style. The *New York Times,* pp. VI–20.

Rabkin, J. G., & Streuning, E. L. (1976). Life events, stress, and illness. *Science, 194,* 1013–1020.

Ramirez, M., III (1984). Assessing and understanding biculturalism-multiculturalism in Mexican-American adults. In J. L. Martinez Jr. & R. H. Mendoza (Eds.), *Chicano Psychology* (2nd ed., pp. 77–93). New York: Academic Press, Inc.

Redfield, R., Linton, R., & Herskovits, M. J. (1936). Memorandum on the study of acculturation. *American Anthropologist, 56,* 973–1002.

Reeves, T., & Bennett, C. (2003). *The Asian and Pacific Islander population in the United States: March 2002.* Retrieved August 27, 2009, from http://www.census.gov/prod/2003pubs/p20-540.pdf.

Rumbaut, R. G., (1995). Vietnamese, Laotian, and Cambodian Americans. In P. G. Min (Ed.), *Asian Americans: Contemporary trends and issues* (pp. 232–270). Thousand Oaks, CA: Sage Publications.

Ryder, A. G., Alden, L. E., & Paulhus, D. L. (2000). Is acculturation unidimensional or bidimensional? A head-to-head comparison in the prediction of personality, self-identity, and adjustment. *Journal of Personality and Social Psychology, 79,* 49–65.

Sandlund, E. S., & Norlander, T. (2000). The effects of Tai Chi Chuan relaxation and exercise on stress responses and well-being: An overview of research. *International Journal of Stress Management, 17,* 139–149.

Segall, M. H., Dasen, P. R., Berry, J. W., & Poortinga, Y. H. (1999). *Human behavior in global perspective: An introduction to cross-cultural psychology* (2nd ed.). Boston: Allyn & Bacon.

Shin, K. R. (1994). Psychosocial predictors of depressive symptoms in Korean-American women in New York City. *Women and Health, 21,* 73–82.

Smart, J. F., & Smart, D. W. (1995). Acculturative stress: The experience of the Hispanic immigrant. *The Counseling Psychologist, 23,* 25–42.

Snowden, L. R., & Cheung, F. H. (1990). Use of inpatient mental health services by members of ethnic minority groups. *American Psychologist, 45,* 347–355.

Spickard, P. R. (1996). *Japanese Americans: The formation and transformation of an ethnic group.* New York: Twayne Publishers.

Sue, D. W. (1994). Asian-American mental health and help-seeking behavior: Comment on Solberg et al. (1994), Tata and Leong (1994), and Lin (1994). *Journal of Counseling Psychology, 41,* 292–295.

Sue, D. W., Capodilupo, C. M., Torino, G. C., Bucceri, J. M., Holder, A. M. B., Nadal, K. L., & Esquilin, M. (2007). Racial microaggressions in everyday life: Implications for clinical practice. *American Psychologist, 62,* 271–286.

Sue, D. W., & Kirk, B. A. (1975). Asian-Americans: Use of counseling and psychiatric services on a college campus. *Journal of Counseling Psychology, 22,* 84–86.

Sue, D. W., & Sue, D. (2003). *Counseling the culturally different: Theory and practice* (4th ed.). New York: John Wiley & Sons, Inc.

Sue, S. (1977). Community mental health services to minority groups: Some optimism, some pessimism. *American Psychologist, 32,* 616–624.

Sue, S., Fujino, D. C., Hu, L., Takeuchi, D. T., & Zane, N. W. S. (1991). Community mental health services for ethnic minority group: A test of the cultural responsiveness hypothesis. *Journal of Consulting and Clinical Psychology, 59,* 533–540.

Sue, S., & McKinney, H. (1975). Asian Americans in the community mental health care system. *American Journal of Orthopsychiatry, 45,* 111–118.

Sue, S., & Morishima, J. K. (1982). *The mental health of Asian Americans.* San Francisco: Jossey-Bass.

Sue, S., & Sue, D. W. (1974). MMPI comparisons between Asian-American and non-Asian students utilizing a student health psychiatric clinic. *Journal of Counseling Psychology, 21,* 423–427.

Sue, S. & Zane, N. (1987). The role of culture and cultural techniques in psychotherapy: A critique and reformulation. *American Psychologist, 42,* 37–45.

Szapocznik, J., & Kurtines, W. M. (1980). Acculturation, biculturalism, and adjustment among Cuban Americans. In A. M. Padilla (Ed.). *Acculturation: Theory, models and some new findings.* Boulder, CO: Westview Press, Inc.

Szapocznik, J., Kurtines, W. M., & Fernandez, T. (1980). Bicultural involvement and adjustment in Hispanic-American youths. *International Journal of Intercultural Relations, 4,* 353–365.

Szapocznik, J., Scopetta, M. A., Kurtines, W., & Aranalde, M. A. (1978). Theory and measurement of acculturation. *Interamerican Journal of Psychology, 12,* 113–120.

Takaki, R. T. (1983). *Pau hana: Plantation life and labor in Hawaii, 1835–1920.* Honolulu: University of Hawaii Press.

Takaki, R. T. (1989). *Strangers from a different shore: A history of Asian Americans.* Boston: Little, Brown and Company.

Tata, S. P., & Leong, F. T. L. (1994). Individualism-collectivism, social-network orientation, and acculturation as predictors of attitudes toward seeking professional psychological help among Chinese Americans. *Journal of Counseling Psychology, 41,* 280–287.

Tsai-Chae, A. H., & Nagata, D. K. (2008). Asian values and perceptions of intergenerational family conflict among Asian American students. *Cultural Diversity and Ethnic Minority Psychology, 14,* 205–214.

Tinloy, M. Y. (1978). Counseling Asian-Americans: A contrast in values. *Journal of Non-White Concerns in Personnel and Guidance, 6,* 71–77.

Tomita, S. K. (1994). The consideration of cultural factors in the research of elder mistreatment with an indepth look at the Japanese. *Journal of Cross-Cultural Gerontology, 9,* 39–52.

Uba, L. (1994). *Asian Americans: Personality Patterns, Identity and Mental Health.* New York: Guilford Press.

U.S. Bureau of the Census. (1990). *Statistical Abstract of the United States: 1990* (110th ed.). Washington, DC: U.S. Government Printing Office.

U.S. Bureau of the Census. (1997). *Statistical Abstract of the United States: 1997* (117th ed.). Washington, DC: U.S. Government Printing Office.

U.S. Bureau of the Census (2002). Race and Hispanic or Latino origin by age and sex for the United States: 2000. Retrieved August 27, 2009, from http://www.census.gov/population/www/cen2000/phc-t08.html.

U.S. Bureau of the Census. (2009). *U.S. interim projections by age, sex, race, and Hispanic origin.* Retrieved August 27, 2009, from http://www.census.gov/ipc/www/usinterimproj/.

U.S. Bureau of the Census. (2009). Asian/Pacific American heritage month: May 2009. Retrieved August 27, 2009, from http://www.census.gov/Press-Release/www/releases/archives/facts_for_features_special_editions/013385.html.

U.S. Department of Health and Human Services. (2001). *Mental health: Culture, race, and ethnicity–A supplement to Mental Health: A report of the Surgeon General.* Rockville, MD: Author.

Walsh, R. (1994). The making of a shaman: Calling training, and culmination. *Journal of Humanistic Psychology, 34,* 7–30.

Walters, G. D. (2001). The Shaman effect in counseling clients with alcohol problems. *Alcoholism Treatment Quarterly, 19,* 31–43.

Wei, W. (1993). *The Asian American movement.* Philadelphia: Temple University Press.

Wijeyesinghe, C. L., Griffin, P., & Love, B. (1997). Racism curriculum design. In M. Adams, L. A. Bell, & P. Griffin (Eds.), *Teaching for diversity and social justice* (pp. 82–110). New York: Routledge.

Wong, B. (1998). *Ethnicity and entrepreneurship: The new Chinese immigrants in the San Francisco bay area.* Boston: Allyn and Bacon.

Wong, P. T. P., & Ujimoto, K. V. (1998). The elderly: Their stress, coping, and mental health. In L. C. Lee & N. W. S. Zane (Eds.), *Handbook of Asian American Psychology.* Thousand Oaks, CA: Sage Publications.

Yi, K. Y. (2000). Shin-byung (divine illness) in a Korean woman. *Culture, Medicine and Psychiatry, 24,* 471–486.

Yoon, I. (1993). *The social origins of Korean immigration to the United States from 1965 to the Present.* Honolulu, Hawaii: East-West Center.

Yoon, I. (1997). *On my own: Korean business and race relations in America.* Chicago: The University of Chicago Press.

Young, K., & Takeuchi, D. T. (1998). Racism. In L. C. Lee & N. W. S. Zane (Eds.), *Handbook of Asian*

American psychology (pp. 401–432). Thousand Oaks, CA: Sage.

Your University of California Online. (2009). Interned Japanese American UC students to receive honorary degrees. Retrieved August 28, 2009, from http://www.universityofcalifornia.edu/youruniversity/story4.html.

Zhang, N., & Dixon, D. N. (2001). Multiculturally responsive counseling: Effects on Asian students' ratings of counselors. *Journal of Multicultural Counseling and Development, 29,* 253–262.

INDEX

A

Abreu, 44
Acculturation theory, 29, 38–44
  contact and participation, 38
  cultural maintenance, 38
  defined, 38
  limitations, 39–40
  theorists, 39
Acculturative Family Distancing (AFD), 30
Acculturative stress, 24, 28–30
Acupuncture, 70
Advocate, 76
African American, 24h
Age range, 6
Ahn, 31
Ailments, 66
Amok, 66
Ancestors, 52
Anger syndrome, 66
Annis, 29
Anxiety, 66
Arizona, 14
Arkansas, 14
Asay, 34
Asian American Racism-Related Stress Inventory
  (AARRSI), 24
Asian Indians, 3, 17
Assimilation, 41
Atkinson, 52, 77
Attitudes
  appreciating, 46
  counseling and, 65
  depreciating, 45–46
  mental health services and, 58–64
  seeking professional psychological help, 60–61

  toward illness, 43
  value dimension and, 44, 47
  willingness to seek counseling for specific problems,
    60–61
  See also Assimilation; Integration;
    Marginalization; Separation
Attitudinal constructs, 60
Authority figures, 50–51
Awareness stage, 45

B

Bennett, 28
Berry, John, 29
Bicultural
Biculturalism, 39, 42
  assessment, 43
  attitudes, 42
  communication ability, 43
  competence, 42–43
  efficacy, 43
  grounding, 43
  knowledge of beliefs and values, 42
  role repertoire, 43
Brenner, 34
Buddhism, 53, 54

C

Caldwell, 77
California, 7, 11, 14
Cambodia, 18
Cambodian-American, 9, 20
Canada, 13
Catholicism, 53–54